SOCIAL PERSPECTIVES ON PREGNANCY AND CHILDBIRTH FOR MIDWIVES, NURSES AND THE CARING PROFESSIONS

Julie Kent

OPEN UNIVERSITY PRESS
Buckingham • Philadelphia

Open University Press
Celtic Court
22 Ballmoor
Buckingham
MK18 1XW

e-mail: enquiries@openup.co.uk
world wide web: http://www.openup.co.uk

and
325 Chestnut Street
Philadelphia, PA 19106, USA

First Published 2000

A catalogue record of this book is available from the British Library

ISBN 0 335 19911 9 (pb)   0 335 19912 7 (hb)

Library of Congress Cataloging-in-Publication Data
Kent. Julie, 1957–
    Social perspectives on pregnancy and childbirth for midwives, nurses and the
caring professions / Julie Kent.
        p.   cm. — (Social science for nurses and the caring professions)
    Includes bibliographical references and index.
    ISBN 0–335–19911–9 (pbk). — ISBN 0–335–19912–7 (hbk)
    1. Pregnancy — Social aspects. 2. Childbirth — Social aspects.
I. Title. II. Series.
RG556.K46 2000
618.2—dc21   99–25146
                                                                        CIP

Typeset by Graphicraft Limited, Hong Kong
Printed and bound in Great Britain by
Marston Book Services Limited, Oxford

SOCIAL PERSPECTIVES ON PREGNANCY AND CHILDBIRTH FOR MIDWIVES, NURSES AND THE CARING PROFESSIONS

SOCIAL SCIENCE FOR NURSES AND THE CARING PROFESSIONS
Series Editor: Professor Pamela Abbott
University of Teesside, Middlesbrough, Cleveland, UK

Current and forthcoming titles

CONTENTS

SERIES EDITOR'S PREFACE

Pregnancy and childbirth are one of the natural events that the majority of women experience. Midwives and nurses play an important role in supporting women during pregnancy and childbirth. However, the medical model that underpins the ways in which medical doctors treat pregnant women, which at best assumes that 'something will go wrong' and at worst treats them as if they were sick, is at odds with women's own understanding. Women understand pregnancy and childbirth as a natural process. Furthermore medical doctors tend to assume that they know best whereas women want to be consulted and give informed consent to any necessary medical intervention. Whereas doctors believe that a satisfactory outcome to pregnancy and childbirth is a well mother and child, women want also to have experience the outcome as pleasurable. The dominance of the medical model and of hospital medicine in Britain and other industralized societies means that that pregnancy and childbirth have become medicalized. However, this medical model has be challenged by midwives and an increasing body of feminist research.

In this book Julie Kent, who is herself a qualified midwife provides a comprehensive overview of the feminist research on pregnancy and childbirth. She also gives an account of her own research. Not only does she provide an account of the literature that is accessible to practitioners but also explores the way in which the findings from the research are relevant to professional practice. This book will not only enable the practitioners understanding but facilitate the further development of evidenced practice.

Pamela Abbott

ACKNOWLEDGEMENTS

Many thanks to all those friends and family who have supported and encouraged me in writing this book. I would especially like to thank those who offered comments on earlier drafts of various chapters including Sue Hatt, Carolyn Britton, Debbie Foster, Kathryn Woodward, Gayle Letherby, Sheila Hunt, Stella Maile, Alison Assister, Tamsin Wilton and Pamela Abbott, who suggested I write this in the first place. Any weaknesses in the finished version are my own. Thanks also to all those at Open University Press, especially Jacinta Evans and Joan Malherbe whose encouragement was much appreciated. Finally I thank Mick for his continuing support, love and care. I would like to dedicate this book to my two sons, Julian and Christopher.

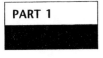

PART 1

THE BIOLOGICAL AND THE SOCIAL

ONE

THE BIOLOGICAL AND THE SOCIAL

Introduction

Becoming pregnant and giving birth are biological events. They involve physiological and physical changes for the woman as the foetus develops and the baby is delivered. While this is a more straightforward process for some women compared to others, even in apparently uncomplicated cases there are complex social processes operating. This book is about those social processes, for in developing an understanding of pregnancy and childbirth we need to go beyond the biological accounts we might find in medical or midwifery texts, or even some of the literature for prospective parents. These kinds of accounts emphasize the physical, physiological and psychological effects of pregnancy and childbirth. They sometimes also include reference to the social implications of becoming a mother or father – how one might adjust to new responsibilities and new feelings. However, they do not attend to the ways in which our understandings of what it is to be pregnant – to be a woman, even – and to give birth are socially produced. So while we cannot deny that biology is important and that physical changes do take place, in this book I aim to show how the very meanings attached to biology, to being a woman, to having a baby, are the products of social processes. These processes occur within specific socio-economic, historical and political contexts. Moreover, the ways in which women experience pregnancy and childbirth are shaped and influenced by these same processes. I shall discuss these later but first I want to consider in more detail the relationship between the biological and the social.

Traditionally there has been a separation between the biological and the social, each being seen as a distinct and separate object of study. Sociologists have been primarily concerned with social and cultural processes and, until more recently, have neglected biology. By seeking to emphasize the social, they have perpetuated a divide between nature/culture and the biological/social that has now been criticized (Scott and Morgan 1993). Efforts by sociologists to avoid **biological reductionism** or suggestions that social and cultural processes are determined by, or products of, biology have resulted in a neglect of the connections between them. However, while this neglect has been seen as widespread in 'malestream/mainstream' social theory, feminist writers have for a long time been concerned with how sex and gender are related.

The major contribution of feminist thought to current debates around biology/bodies has been recognized (Frank 1991a; Scott and Morgan 1993). Biological **sex differences** between men and women have, historically, been emphasized. But increasingly biology came to be seen as an inadequate explanation of how and why women and men are treated differently or experience their lives differently. Feminists drew attention to **gender differences**, arguing that differences between 'men' and 'women' were **socially constructed**. The notion that there are irreducible differences between the sexes has now been discredited and, more recently, the connections between the biological (sex) and the social (gender) have been seen as extremely complex.

Rather than seeing the biological as separate from the social, the two may be seen as closely intertwined. Biological 'sex' may itself be seen as socially constituted, for even in biological terms the differences between 'men' and 'women' are not clear-cut. So social divisions do not simply arise from biological differences; instead, we need to rethink the relationship between the biological and the social. Recently, while feminists have always been interested in women's bodies, the need for a sociology of the body has been identified.

In advocating a sociology of the body and increased attention to biology, Scott and Morgan (1993) show that exploring the connections between the biological and the social leads to a questioning of the very separation of these two spheres. For according to them, sociology enables us to open up 'biology or nature' to examine how it is culturally and historically created. Therefore, according to this view, biology is not the base upon which social and cultural processes operate; rather, the constitution of bodies/biology is itself socially produced. The ways in which we 'see' bodies or understand biology is at issue. Moreover the earlier traditions of sociology which emphasized rationality and methodologies that reinforced a mind/body or culture/nature, social/biological split may be linked to the concerns of **modernism** and a particular historical moment. In contrast, Scott and Morgan (following Turner 1992), suggest that a revisioning of the sociological project to include and attend to biology – or more specifically, *bodies* – is necessary. This has important consequences since it both legitimates new forms of knowledge and places bodily experiences at the centre of sociological inquiry. For it is bodies, as part of systems of action (Giddens 1991) which work, know, have sex, and – more specifically – female bodies which become pregnant and give birth. In other words, bodies are the site of human action in the social world.

It follows that to suggest quite simply that pregnancy and childbirth are 'natural' events in the lives of many women the world over (a biological fact) tells us very little. Instead I want to examine in this book how these events are historically and culturally produced. In so doing I aim to question the 'naturalness' of pregnancy and consider how, in contemporary society, becoming pregnant is a complex event which merits sociological attention. How do women become pregnant and why? Why do some women choose not to get pregnant or find they cannot? In what ways does becoming pregnant relate to a set of social relationships that might vary between women?

Ann Oakley's early studies, *Becoming a Mother* (1979) and *Women Confined: Towards a Sociology of Childbirth* (1980) show how the biological and the social are interconnected. We see how the social conditions of women shape and influence their experience of pregnancy, childbirth and motherhood. More recently, in her study *Social Support and Motherhood* (1992), Oakley demonstrates how the social has biological effects by examining how the birth weight of the baby and the woman's own health are influenced by class inequalities, **material deprivation**, stress and other social factors. According to Oakley (1992: 327): 'the provision of sympathetic, listening support through continuity of care, which is what women have been requiring whenever anyone has thought to ask them, is a more effective way to promote their health and that of their babies than most of the medical interventions carried out in the name of antenatal "care"'.

Moreover, Oakley argues (as do many others) that women, or rather *midwives*, are best placed to act as carers (or sympathetic listeners) for pregnant women because of the 'culture of gender, and the differences in professional training and ideology between midwives and obstetricians' (Oakley 1992: 327). So why is this? What do we mean by professional **ideology**? What are the differences in professional training between midwives and obstetricians that are so significant? What does becoming a mother mean today? Has anything changed, or is it likely to? Certainly these are some of the questions that Oakley's work addresses and they continue to be of concern to many other writers.

My intention here, therefore, is to show how a range of issues relating to pregnancy and childbirth today may be understood with reference to social theories. For as soon as we begin to step outside a simple biological account and to explore the social we need the conceptual tools to describe and discuss those issues.

Contemporary issues relating to pregnancy and childbirth

The issues of today may frequently only be understood with reference to the past. Historical accounts therefore of the medical care of pregnant women (Oakley 1986), of midwives and medical men (Donnison 1977), of reproductive medicine (Pfeffer 1993), and of the history of sexuality (Foucault 1979, 1985, 1990; Hawkes 1996) will all be relevant to this discussion. But first let me outline some of the key issues and some central debates of concern.

Of primary concern is the extent to which women have control over their own bodies. In recent years there has been increased debate, particularly influenced by feminist theory, about the ways in which women's bodies are loved, oppressed, exploited, abused and controlled. These concerns arise in relation to the experiences of women as workers, mothers, wives and lovers. They are also important in analysing or discussing sexual harassment, sex, rape and violence against women, pornography, health/illness and indeed pregnancy and childbirth. So one of the issues I shall address later is: should women have greater control over their pregnancy and childbirth than currently and if so how may this be achieved?

Issues of control and choice are frequently raised in discussions of reproductive technologies and the new genetics. For as scientific and technological developments result in the introduction of new diagnostic procedures, therapies and treatments, some people believe that they present greater choice and control for women. The introduction of contraceptive devices and most notably 'the pill' was heralded as bringing greater freedom for women and enhanced control over their reproductive lives. Yet others argue that these freedoms and increased choice have other costs and that the benefits are not all one way. Rather, the interests of capitalists and patriarchs (men) are served by these same technologies. Indeed the very concept of choice is hotly contested for it is sometimes assumed that women choose, or make decisions about their lives, in a vacuum. However, if we examine the conditions under which those choices are made, the pressures to act in one way, rather than another, begin to come into view.

- In whose interest are the new reproductive technologies being developed?
- Can women benefit from them or is the cost too high?

Linked to these technologies and the position of women in contemporary society are questions about what it means to be a mother in that society. Since techniques such as in vitro fertilization (IVF) and donor insemination shape new social relationships between donors and recipients, the doctor and client, surrogate mothers and adoptive mothers, the very idea of 'motherhood' has become problematized in new ways. In addition, since many women work and have families, changes in work practices and changes in the family are also important.

The role of the doctor and other health professionals, especially midwives, is also of interest because of the connections between knowledge and professional power. As Oakley (1989) and others have argued the professional domains and demarcations between obstetrician and midwife lead to conflicts around and over women's bodies (Witz 1992).

- Why is professional power important?
- What are its sources and its consequences?
- What are the connections between knowledge and power?

Once pregnant, a woman's body changes shape, takes on different forms and is seen in a different light.

- What images of pregnant bodies do we see? How are they used?
- How do women themselves view pregnancy and motherhood?

I will explore these questions in order to show how images and cultural **representations** shape what we think about pregnancy. These representations mediate our view of what both being a woman and being pregnant means. In medical practice, visualizing the female body has been important for diagnostic purposes and the development of new imaging technologies is associated with the construction of the foetus as a new patient (subject) distinct from its mother.

The links between sex, gender and sexuality are dynamic and changing. I aim to develop an understanding of sexual identities, how sexuality is organized in contemporary society (Weeks 1981, 1985, 1986) and how this relates to pregnancy and childbirth. I will explore how sex, reproduction and marriage have been tied together and the extent to which being a 'real woman' means becoming a mother. This then will assist in analysing why lesbian women might want to have children without a relationship with a man, and how commonly **heterosexist** assumptions underpin the provision of maternity care in the UK. The marginalization of homosexual men in society and the links between being male, masculinity and fatherhood will also be discussed.

Sociological perspectives – theoretical tools

By suggesting that the issues identified above might usefully be explored from a sociological perspective I mean to demonstrate how a range of theoretical tools from sociology may be applied. In effect this means that in each of the following chapters I draw on an area of sociological thought. There are however important links between each chapter and four key concepts running throughout the book: *knowledge, power, identity* and the *body*. I shall explore the links between these concepts, however, each of the four parts concentrates on a specific concept. In Part 1 I draw attention to different types of *knowledge* and ways of knowing. In Part 2, via a discussion of the midwifery profession, I examine the connections between knowledge and *power* in the workplace and in education settings. The focus of Part 3 is *identity* – how women are seen as mothers and how sexual identities are constructed. The construction of identities is linked to knowledge and power but also to bodies, so in Part 4 the ways in which women's *bodies* are represented and the significance of new reproductive technologies for women is discussed. In order to develop an understanding of pregnancy and childbirth from a sociological perspective it is important to get to grips with these central concepts and the relationships between them (see Box 1.1).

Box 1.1 Key concepts in this book	
KNOWLEDGE	POWER
(Part 1)	(Part 2)
IDENTITY	BODY
(Part 3)	(Part 4)

Ways of knowing

So far I have outlined how biology and sociology have focused on different objects of study and used different methods or ways of knowing. In Chapter 2, in order to analyse recent policy developments in maternity service provision as set out in *Changing Childbirth* (Department of Health 1993), I will be using theoretical ideas from the sociology of knowledge. This will enable me to examine the knowledge claims of doctors and midwives who are frequently seen to present competing approaches to childbirth. Those approaches rest on competing and often conflicting **paradigms** and I shall explore the view that the scientific paradigm (of medicine/obstetrics) is increasingly under threat from 'alternative' approaches to childbirth.

In many discussions of reproduction we find that the scientific paradigm characterizes the work of obstetricians or doctors, while midwives are seen as women-centred, as 'guardians of the normal', promoting a view of childbirth as a natural and normal process. Oakley (1986) and other writers (for example, Katz Rothman 1982) describe a process of **medicalization**, whereby obstetricians have increased their control over women receiving maternity services. I shall explore this debate and show how a simple polarization of medical versus midwifery models is inadequate to illuminate women's experience of childbirth. Critics of the medicalization thesis argue that it implies that women have been duped. An overemphasis on medicalization leads to a view that women accept medical definitions of their bodily experiences and obstetric care without question (Williams and Calnan 1996). Clearly this isn't the case for women have been active in seeking alternative approaches to maternity care (Garcia *et al.* 1990). At the same time the idea that midwives represent a completely different approach to pregnancy and childbirth is also misleading, because many midwives collude with, and support a medicalized view of childbirth (Bryar 1995). In addition, institutionalized patterns of working provide them with both professional status and relative autonomy. While some midwives prefer to work independently – that is, outside the National Health Service (NHS) – and many wish to promote greater continuity of care, they are not always a majority. These issues will be the focus of Chapter 2.

The professionals

Professional politics in an education setting is the subject of Chapter 3. Since there have recently been significant changes in the provision of midwifery education these will be discussed with reference to ideas of **'professionalization'** and 'demarcationary strategies' (Witz 1992) between the nursing, midwifery and medical professions. In the case of midwives it seems that these changes have been seen both as representing a fundamental threat to their professional or social identity as midwives and as an opportunity to strengthen professional power (Kent 1995, 1999). For some time now sociologists have developed analyses of what constitutes a profession, the sources of professional power, professional interests, professionals' roles as agents of social control and of the state. These ideas will be seen as relevant to understanding the midwifery profession and what it means to be a midwife today. This in turn is important for assessing the contribution midwives make in caring for women during pregnancy and childbirth.

In England, midwifery education has recently established links with higher education through the development of diploma and degree courses (Kent *et al.* 1994). These links, and the increasing emphasis on academic input and theoretical knowledge related to practice, signal a move away from an apprenticeship model of training. The implications for midwifery practice are still being assessed (Kent *et al.* 1994; Eraut *et al.* 1995; Gerrish *et al.* 1996a; Phillips *et al.* 1996; Fraser *et al.* 1997). I suggest that it is possible to see these changes as attempts to reinforce **credentialism** and **occupational closure** and as part of professionalizing strategies. Like the nursing profession, midwives are increasingly concerned to identify a knowledge base for their practice that is distinct and legitimates what they do. However, they appear to be caught in a dilemma, for while some want to reject medicalized views of pregnancy and childbirth, they also aspire to the status of a profession. At the same time as wanting to express the ways in which they are different from doctors they work, perhaps unintentionally, towards becoming like them. With respect to nurses, midwives are also caught in a paradox. In so far as they allow similarities between them and nurses to be highlighted – by, for example, joint training programmes such as Project 2000 – they gain political power through collaboration with a large and more powerful group. However, this very collaboration for many signals a weakening of midwives' position, a dilution of their statutory responsibilities, greater difficulty in asserting a view of pregnancy and childbirth as normal, healthy and natural, and a weakening of their claim to be independent practitioners. For midwives these are important distinctions since nurses, in their view, are primarily concerned with sickness and ill health and are subordinate to doctors.

In Chapter 4 an understanding of the **division of labour** between midwives and doctors will be developed. Historical accounts of the development of these two professions are seen to have resulted in a sexual division of labour. The gendering of work and in particular 'care' work as 'women's work' will be examined. This will lead to a discussion of how what midwives do is sometimes seen as an extension of what women do 'naturally'. According to such a view the position of male midwives is particularly ambiguous and needs some explanation but so too does the relationship between midwives and the women they 'care' for.

I shall examine the claim made by midwives to be 'with women' and how, when caring for pregnant and labouring women, midwives frequently align their own interests with those of the woman. However, this emancipatory discourse needs closer consideration, for in what sense are the interests of midwives and women the same? Indeed much of the literature on the professions suggests that professionals act in their own interests at the expense of clients, so are midwives very different, and if so, in what ways? I argue that midwives do seem to deliver the kind of care women want for themselves but, at the same time, claims to represent the interests of women, in practice, enable midwives to strengthen their professional status and identity.

Constructing identities

Sociological approaches to the family are important for exploring the issues around motherhood. Becoming a mother commonly implies that new responsibilities, new duties and a different role for the woman will follow. The nature and form of these can only be understood in the context of the set of relationships where mothers are situated. Many of these relationships have traditionally constituted 'a family'. However, it is frequently suggested that traditional families are far less common today, that many women who are mothers are lone parents through separation, divorce, desertion (as in Ireland), or choice. The very concept of a family is problematic and the position of women within one is particularly so. Through this discussion of families, in Chapter 5, ideologies of 'mother-hood' will be uncovered, and this will assist in developing an understanding of the implications of becoming a mother for a woman's identity.

The relationship between caring and being a mother will be examined and this will be elaborated with reference to continuing debate about the division of labour in the home. Women, especially mothers, have always been identified with caring for children and carrying out domestic labour. Mothers' experiences relate to the relationship between the private sphere of 'home' and the public sphere of 'work'. In modern Britain women are more likely to be older when they become mothers, compared to their own mothers, and also more likely to be working and looking after children. Recent attempts to encourage lone mothers to enter paid employment will also be discussed. The evidence suggests then that there are a number of changes in both the pattern of childbirth and the experience of becoming a mother which need explaining. A sociological perspective assists in understanding how far the nuclear family, or at least a revised version of it, continues to be seen as central to contemporary western society.

The formation of sexual and gendered identities is the subject of Chapter 6. In this discussion I will examine in more detail what we mean by 'identity' and the organization of sexuality. I shall consider the links between sex, gender and sexuality, how different types of bodies are produced and how sexual desires and sexual activity are regulated. Rather than seeing identity as a fixed and stable concept tied to biology, I shall argue that it is constantly being produced in different settings through the discursive ordering of a social world. Sexual identities are situated historically in the development of the 'civilized', 'modern' world where the sexuality of women and homosexual men became defined as particularly problematic. The dominance of hetereosexuality in a **'masculinist'** culture is seen as tying together sex, reproduction and marriage which in turn marginalizes lesbian women (and homosexual men), disabled women, lone mothers and women who are involuntarily childless or child-free. Public policy relating to fertility control, abortion and infertility treatment and the medicalization of pregnancy and childbirth is understood in the context of dominant ideas about sex and sexuality. I suggest that underpinning the provision of maternity and health services is a traditional and unitary view of women.

Chapter 6 shows how **discourses**, bodies and institutions intersect, producing gender and sexual identities. While the focus of this book is women's bodies I also consider here the relationship of men to father-hood. This requires a discussion of 'masculinities' – that is, how the gen-der identities of men are constructed in a hierarchy which positions white, heterosexual middle-class men in a powerful position. I conclude that an understanding of the formation of sexual and gender identities and the regulation of sexuality could usefully enhance the health care practices of nurses, midwives, doctors and others.

Women's bodies

In Chapter 7, by outlining the central debates surrounding the growth of reproductive technologies, I will draw on sociological perspectives of sci-ence and technology. This points to questions about how technologies are shaped and produced and the kinds of social relationships which form around them. While avoiding a **technologically determinist** view (the idea that technologies necessarily produce one set of relationships rather than any other) I will examine the view that those relationships deter-mine the shape and form of the technologies. A central issue is whether these technologies are themselves neutral and benign, or if, as already suggested above, they serve particular interests. Moreover, at the centre are women's bodies that may be seen as sites of struggle and conflict, where knowledge and power intersect. While these technologies are used to act upon women, women themselves appear to be active in appropriat-ing them. Women may be seen not just as passive victims, but as agents seeking to gain control over their lives. In the context of new information about the links between genes (or genetic markers) and diseases, women are faced with particularly complex decisions. These will be discussed and the role of genetic counsellors examined.

In Chapter 8 my attention turns to the ways in which women's bodies, or more specifically women's pregnant bodies, are visually represented. This includes a look at diagnostic imaging and the images produced of the mother and foetus. My interest here is in how the **representation** of pregnant bodies in these images shapes and influences what being preg-nant means. These meanings are culturally produced and situate a preg-nant woman in specific ways – for example, as a container of the foetus, as a young woman, as a consumer of baby products. The ways in which these images are used reveals a great deal about social attitudes to preg-nancy. In fact, when we begin to look for images of pregnant women, we find that they are not as widely available as we might expect. In a sense, being pregnant means being hidden – invisible. The experiences of preg-nant women tell us that the visibility of their pregnancy is indeed a source of embarrassment for them and others, and not easily accommo-dated within everyday settings. By examining how women's pregnant bodies have been visualized in art, in medicine and in popular culture I aim to reach a better understanding of the connection between the **sym-bolic** and the **material** aspects of having a female body and being pregnant.

Throughout this book I explore the issues from sociological perspectives which are informed by feminist theory. This is intentional since for me it is the only way I can make sense of those issues and theorize them. My own experiences as a woman and a mother also inform this discussion and shape my agenda in writing this book. Indeed in many ways this is a reflective essay since my own experiences of being pregnant and giving birth occurred over 20 years ago and now, as my sons enter their adult life, I am able to reassess what being a mother means.

Finally, in Chapter 9 I suggest how health professionals and others might use the ideas discussed in this book. My aim is to suggest an agenda for bringing about change in practical ways. Theory and practice are interlinked, and by developing a sociological (theoretical) understanding of pregnancy and childbirth, practical steps can be taken to improve the position of women, the services provided and health care practices. This book is intended to show that by applying social and feminist theory to the issues and questions raised, midwives, nurses and others may become better equipped to think critically about the kind of future we want for ourselves. We might then be able to assess whether new technologies, new ways of working and new ways of being are more beneficial to us all.

Summary

- Chapter 1 describes the main purpose and organization of this book. The book aims to show how the biological and social aspects of pregnancy and childbirth are interconnected. In order that nurses, midwives and the caring professions may develop a better understanding of the social aspects, the aim is to explore key issues and questions (see Box 1.2) using sociological perspectives. This means using a range of social theories and sociological concepts. Each subsequent chapter therefore draws on existing work in different areas of sociology. The implications of adopting a sociological perspective of pregnancy and childbirth for health care practice will also be discussed.

Box 1.2 Some key questions explored in this book

- Should women have greater control over their pregnancy and childbirth than currently and if so how may this be achieved?
- In whose interest are the new reproductive technologies being developed?
- Can women benefit from them or is the cost too high?
- Why is professional power important?
- What are its sources and its consequences?
- What are the connections between knowledge and power?
- What images of pregnant bodies do we see? How are they used?
- How do women themselves view pregnancy and motherhood?

TWO

WHO KNOWS BEST? COMPETING APPROACHES TO CHILDBIRTH

Introduction

There is a well-documented history of changes in childbirth which, from a sociological perspective, may be understood as a continuing conflict between women, doctors and midwives. Essentially this is a conflict about who knows best, about different views of pregnancy and childbirth. It is also about the ability of different groups to exercise power, to influence and shape the kind of services provided. Analysis of these conflicts will help practitioners to understand the social and political processes that impact on the formation of maternity policies and the organization of maternity care in the UK.

In the 1990s this conflict was explicitly recognized by the British government in its policy document *Changing Childbirth* (Department of Health 1993). Reporting on a conference convened in 1993 a consensus statement read: 'There is no place for professional rivalries which only hinder the provision of good maternity services, and it is clear that tensions do exist in some places' (Department of Health 1993: 106). This followed the earlier report of the House of Commons Select Committee in 1992 that said, 'much of what we heard appeared to be concerned with which group should have control over the maternity services'. The committee also said, 'differences of opinion in this area appear to stem from divergent philosophies of the management of pregnancy and childbirth between what has frequently been described to us as a "medical" and a "non-medical" view of the process' (House of Commons Select Committee 1992, para. 175).

For years sociologists have been writing about these tensions and exploring the divergent philosophies that underlie them. By summarizing these earlier accounts my aim is to examine the extent to which proposed changes in childbirth policy might be expected to resolve some of these tensions. Are we witnessing a transformation in the power relations between these groups and a shift in the knowledge/power nexus? In order to answer this question I shall first outline the development of maternity services in the NHS and the rising influence of medical knowledge. The shape and form of maternity services will be linked to the position of doctors in the NHS but explained with reference to the work of social theorists such as Weber, Foucault and Turner. I shall contrast this medical model of pregnancy and childbirth with a midwifery model. The history of midwifery predates the medical profession but in modern society it has been argued that midwifery knowledge has been undervalued. The position of midwives may be explained by understanding the relationship between knowledge and power and a gender hierarchy. This hierarchy also helps to explain attitudes to women's own experiences and views of pregnancy. I shall consider whether the policy changes that are taking place are likely to reshape the institutional arrangements for maternity care and the relationships between doctors, midwives and women. These debates are important for health care professionals since they explain how broader historical, social and political processes shape the scope of professional practice.

The stated intention of government is to improve maternity services in England. In *Changing Childbirth* (Department of Health 1993) women are expected to have a greater say in the care they receive. However, the extent to which this marks a radical change in the way in which pregnancy and childbirth is viewed is an open question. Changes in care are being sought elsewhere too. The evidence from other countries, for example Ireland, suggests that changes in the availability of community-based midwifery services are likely to be a long time in coming. Maternity care there continues to be centralized and dominated by medical professionals (O'Connor 1992, 1995). In poorer countries the standard of care for pregnant and parturient women is often ineffective and many women suffer ill health through a lack of care. According to Lesley Doyal 'a WHO study in the early 1980s found that in many countries less than 40 per cent of women had seen a qualified health worker during their pregnancy' (Doyal 1995: 132). As Doyal points out, better access to obstetric care has contributed to making childbirth safer for women in rich countries. Though it was by no means the only factor, since improved nutrition and sanitary conditions were also significant: 'the importance of these developments for women's health and well-being cannot be overestimated' (p. 133). If this is the case what is at issue here, and why has there been such widespread dissatisfaction with maternity services in the UK?

The medicalization of life

In her well-known book *The Captured Womb*, Ann Oakley gives an historical account of the **medicalization** of pregnancy. She argues that there were two stages to medicalization. First, in the eighteenth century, was the idea of pregnancy as 'natural' when 'medical practitioners upheld a paradigm of pregnancy which decisively appealed to *nature* as the arbiter of its proper management' (Oakley 1986: 12). Advice and information given to women at that time she suggests, was not distinguished from obstetric knowledge. However, by systematizing women's experiences the medical practitioner *appropriated* knowledge of pregnancy and began to redefine it as technical and medical expertise. Later, pregnancy became defined as pathological and came increasingly under the control of the state and health professionals. This enabled the health professional to become established as the expert. I shall argue in Chapter 3 that both midwives and medical men established themselves in this way though the basis of their claims to expertise will be seen as different. First I will consider the 'medical model' of pregnancy that characterizes maternity care in twentieth-century Britain (and the USA) and then contrast it with what I call the 'midwifery model'.

Ways of knowing

The rise of medical power and increased medicalization of life is linked, in sociological accounts, to the **secularization** of society and the development of modern capitalist societies (Turner 1995). It is part of a broader social, historical and political process. As Turner suggests we need a sociology of knowledge approach to the development of medicine for we cannot take medical categories of disease, or definitions of health and illness simply as objective criteria. Although medicine commonly makes such a claim, and asserts that medical knowledge is objective, neutral and unbiased, for sociologists this is deeply problematic. Instead, medical knowledge is itself regarded as socially and culturally produced for 'it is simply the case that different types of society have different types of disease and different approaches to therapy; these variations are the products of culture and social organisation' (Turner 1995: 18). Moreover, medical theories change over time. Consequently a theory of knowledge (**epistemology**) which sets the scientist or doctor apart from that which he or she studies, which insists that the disease is an **independent variable**, a separate entity (with an **ontology** that is distinct), glosses over the ways in which knowledge of the disease is socially produced. It is for this reason that medical practice, and more specifically the medical model of pregnancy, has been severely criticized.

By providing a detailed historical account of the changes in knowledge about pregnancy through history, Oakley (1986) illustrates the ways in which knowledge is socially and culturally produced (see Box 2.1). She shows how changing attitudes to antenatal care were associated with the **scientization** and medicalization of pregnancy. New technologies and techniques for observing and measuring, or assessing, pregnancy effectively took control from the woman and repositioned her as a tool, or artefact, within the **technical rationality** of the physician.

Box 2.1   A history of medical technologies used in obstetrics
(material drawn from Oakley 1986)

1808   Obstetrician in the USA claims to have 'discovered' effects of ergot for inducing labour
1882   Ceasarian sections successfully performed in Germany
1908   X-rays used to examine pregnant women
1930s   Three popular methods of inducing labour in use: ARM (artificial rupture of membranes); drug therapy; and mechanical dilation of cervix, though techniques for inducing labour date back to the nineteenth century
        Forceps and episiotomy routine procedure for breech delivery in the UK
1931   Bode records electrical activity of human uterus during labour
1950s   Cervical 'cerclage' to prevent premature delivery
1957   First ultrasound of pregnant woman – ultrasound screening becomes routine in 1970s
1960s   Electro-foetal monitoring during labour
        Drug therapy to prevent preterm labour including hormone treatments
        Titration of oxytocin drugs for induction of labour
1970s   Fetoscopy
1978   Amniocentesis screening test developed
        First IVF baby (Louise Brown) born

Note: dates here are approximate for, as Oakley says, the origins of these technologies and practices often predate the time when obstetricians claimed to have discovered their value in obstretrics.

The medical model of pregnancy has been seen to have certain characteristics and following from this, effects which have led to dissatisfaction with maternity services. Closely tied in with theories of medical knowledge are theories of the body. Medicine is specifically concerned with the 'treatment' of bodies and obstetrics, as a branch of medicine, with women's pregnant bodies. The principle methods used to study the body have been observation and experimentation. A process of **objectification** occurs where the personhood of the body is ignored; the body is seen as an object of analysis rather than a thinking, feeling human being. At the same time there is a hierarchy of knowledge as the observer's knowledge is assumed to be the correct one while the views or experiences of the person observed are largely discounted. Accordingly, pregnant women have described feelings of **alienation** and **marginalization** as they have been treated as objects on a conveyer belt, a case or even just a number. The widely accepted practice of **randomized controlled trials** in medical and obstetric research reinforces the aim to control subjects in the research and allocate them a number (see Box 2.2). **Universalism** is also characteristic in so far as all bodies are treated the same, assumed to have the same basic attributes that can be expected to respond similarly under the same conditions and therefore to which findings can be universally applied.

> ### Box 2.2 A randomized controlled trial – a method explained
>
> The population to be sampled is assigned a number and then randomly selected for the study. (In some studies samples of matched pairs are selected.) In a controlled trial there is an intervention group and a control group. Those selected to take part in the study are allocated to one of these groups. Those in the intervention group will receive some kind of intervention or treatment that is being tested (e.g. drug therapy or social support). Those in the control group will not receive the treatment or intervention. The results of each group will be compared in order to assess the effects of the intervention. In a blind trial the researchers do not know who is in the control group or the intervention group. This is expected to minimize unintended effects of selection.
>
> This method is common in medical and midwifery research but generally considered less appropriate for social research. Critics of the approach argue that it is unethical to withhold treatment which is expected to be beneficial from those in the control group and also that the manipulation of persons in this way is unjustified. It is for this reason that Ann Oakley (1992: 117) asked 'who's afraid of the randomised controlled trial?'

Another feature of the medical model is **reductionism** when the focus of study and interest is narrowed or reduced to physical and physiological processes, neglecting social, political and economic factors. This reductionism has failed to account for the relationship between the biological and the social, embodiment and society, and is underpinned by a **methodological individualism**. The medical model is also **mechanistic**.

The body as machine has been an important metaphor for developing medical knowledge and practice. A systems approach to the body has predominated in the modern era and medicine has focused on malfunctions understood as a breakdown in these systems. This has emphasized continuity and unchanging aspects of bodily function. According to some critics this has perpetuated a masculinist model which is unable to take account of the constantly changing and cyclical pattern of women's bodily experiences, other than to pathologize them. Pregnancy, as a state of change and flux, therefore was constituted as pathological and rather than being left to 'nature' women have been increasingly encouraged to seek the assistance and advice of expert medical practitioners. As Oakley says, 'science or reason' supports the approach of the obstetrician (Oakley 1989, 1992). Claims to knowledge made by obstetricians were contingent on the broader acceptance and legitimation of science and scientific methods in modern industrial society. What is also interesting is the way in which modern health care systems have developed which incorporate this scientific approach by, for example, having regular medical appointments during pregnancy and screening programmes.

Institutionalization of maternity care – the NHS

A television documentary reporting on 50 years of maternity care (BBC 1997) showed how, since the inception of the NHS the organization of maternity services has dehumanized and controlled the ways in which women experience pregnancy and childbirth. Women interviewed for the programme recalled being told very little about what was happening to them, feeling they were on a conveyor belt and that care was organized in a way which was designed to be convenient for the doctor. Before the NHS many women had enjoyed the care of a midwife in their own homes where they had given birth. From the 1920s there was an increased emphasis on hospital birth that was accelerated by the setting up of the NHS. Hospital birth increasingly became characterized as impersonal, threatening and often frightening.

This raises questions about how far the medical model of pregnancy and childbirth is necessarily tied to particular organizational forms. I have already mentioned that medicalization is commonly linked to the development of modern industrial societies. Following Weber's theory of the **rationalization** and **bureaucratization** of social life, the founding of the NHS seems consistent with this (Perry 1997). It is a highly bureaucratized and centralized service. There are therefore a number of parallel processes that underpin the position of doctors and midwives today.

Prior to the inception of the NHS there was competition between doctors and midwives for patients. Increasingly, pregnancy came to be seen by the medical profession as a sphere of practice for them. Medical care of pregnant women was a lucrative business and an important source of revenue for doctors but for poor women who could not afford the doctors' fees the midwife was in heavy demand. As we shall see in Chapter 4 the ability of doctors to define their sphere of practice and limit the areas of midwifery work requires analysis of both gender and class relations (Donnison 1977; Witz 1992). It has been argued that the medical profession were better organized and had close links and shared interests with key decision makers, so they were able to shape the organization of health care. During the eighteenth and nineteenth centuries the rise of medical power increasingly threatened the position of midwives though many women continued to depend on midwifery care.

The influential social theorist, Michel Foucault (see Box 2.3), highlights the connection between knowledge and power by linking medicine to social control. For him, and subsequently many other sociologists such as Turner, the development of the hospital, or clinic, and the asylum are directly tied to the rise of medical knowledge and practice. Turner sees parallels between Foucault and Weber in so far as they were both concerned with aspects of the regulation of the body and self (Turner 1992: 19). He connects medicalization, secularization and rationalization, though he has been criticized for not making these connections clear. Drawing on Foucauldian ideas Turner argues that much of the application of scientific medicine was concerned with the production of a healthy labour force and this rationalization of labour is a feature of capitalism achieved through the disciplining and regulating of bodies or what Bentham called **'panopticism'** (Porter 1998). The hospital provides a centralized location and physical space for the control and **surveillance** of bodies by medical practitioners. The Nightingale ward was a standard design for a hospital ward in every hospital, with beds down either side and the nurses' station at one end (Hunt and Symonds 1995). In *The Birth of the Clinic*, Foucault (1973) described how the medical gaze defines the 'normal' and 'abnormal'. This process of categorization and surveillance also had a moral function:

> Medical practice in our time clearly does have a *moral* function especially in response to AIDS and IVF programmes for unmarried single women, but these moral functions are typically disguised and they are ultimately legitimised by an appeal to scientific rather than religious authority . . . thus in Foucauldian terminology, medicine occupies a social space left by the erosion of religion.
>
> (Turner 1992: 22, emphasis added)

I shall return to the moral function of medical practice and Foucault's ideas later, in Chapter 6. Here it is important to understand the status which scientific medical knowledge came to have in modern, secular society.

In examining the creation of the NHS Klein argues that 'there was nothing inevitable about the final shape of the NHS in 1948' (1983: 26) and even though there was a consensus about the aims of policy there was conflict about the means by which it could be accomplished. According to Klein, the ability of the medical profession to influence and shape services was unique and gave them clinical autonomy and a role in running the NHS. So why was this and how can it be explained? The ability of medical practitioners to influence and shape the development of maternity services rested on the logic of bringing women to the experts. At the

Box 2.3   Foucault – a key thinker

Michel Foucault was a French philosopher, historian and social theorist who died in 1984. His ideas have been very influential though he does have his critics. One of his principal concerns was to give an historical account of knowledge or what he called 'regimes of truth' in the modern world. By tracing the development of ideas in society he developed a discourse theory of knowledge. In his work, knowledge and power are intimately connected through what he calls discourse. The concept of discourse is much debated but may be seen as the form which knowledge takes. Crucially, discourse constructs both the object of knowledge and the subject, the known and the knower and both are shaped by historical and material conditions.

In Foucault's view there are no essential or fixed structures underpinning social life, waiting to be discovered. He also argues that there is no fixed subject, individuals do not simply exist independently of the world around them and interpret it. Instead his work examines the conditions under which complex relations of power produce knowers and knowledge. The effects of discourse are to construct relationships of power. It is the power to define what is 'true' which (re)produces inequalities between social groups and maintains social divisions. These inequalities are linked to institutional forms such as the family, the hospital, the asylum, government. His study of medicine in the modern world examines how doctors became agents of social control with moral authority, disciplining and regulating bodies. Their authority was produced and legitimated by the discourse of science and scientific medical knowledge which characterizes the modern world. The study of the human body in medicine constructed a certain view of what it means to be human, a view which was primarily derived from the study of the anatomy of human corpses. Medical discourse developed systems and rules for classifying features of human bodies and categories of disease but the ability of doctors to know these things must be seen as historically contingent.

Foucault's works include:
The Birth of the Clinic (1973) and *The History of Sexuality* (vols 1–3) (1979, 1985, 1990).

Introductions to Foucault's work include:
Dreyfus, H. and Rabinow, P. (1982) *Michel Foucault: Beyond Structuralism and Hermeneutics.* Brighton: Harvester Press.
McHoul, A. and Grace, W. (1993) *A Foucault Primer: Discourse, Power and the Subject.* London: University College London Press.
Porter, S. (1998) *Social Theory and Nursing Practice.* London: Macmillan.

same time this was legitimated by, and reinforced, their authority as experts. It also enabled them to create a clinical environment where sufficient numbers of pregnant women were available for the practice of obstetrical techniques that increasingly became dependent on large amounts of capital expenditure for high-tech equipment. The training of doctors (and midwives) was seen as requiring a central pool of women to practise on (see Chapter 3).

Specialization and an increasingly complex division of labour between health professionals contributed to the fragmentation of 'the patient'. Different parts of a woman's body and different 'stages' of the pregnancy became designated within the area of expertise of different health workers (Lewis 1980). So, for example, in the new NHS antenatal care was often the responsibility of the general practitioner (GP) or community midwife, with occasional visits to the hospital-based antenatal clinic for check-ups by the radiographer, obstetrician, and hospital midwife. In this way both the organization of care and the experience of being pregnant became more fragmented.

The foetus also was constructed as a new patient for the obstetrician, one that they had only acquired knowledge of by the use of new technologies such as X-rays, ultrasound (in the 1960s) and fibreoptics or fetoscopy (in the early 1970s) (Oakley 1986). This surveillance of the foetus extended the techniques of surveillance applied to the mother and therefore the scope of influence and control that obstetricians had over the mother and baby. It also created the possibility of seeing the foetus as separate from the mother. This, as we shall see in Chapter 7, had important implications for a redefinition of women as subjects, and their rights with respect to their bodies. It also informs the debate around abortion and infertility treatments (Petchesky 1986, 1987; Pfeffer 1993).

A Foucauldian analysis of the connections between knowledge and power therefore enables us to see the development of obstetrics as a way of extending control over, and regulating pregnant bodies. This control and regulation occurs through the construction of a medicalized discourse, or language, used to talk about pregnancy which produces specific practices around the 'management' of pregnant women. 'Active management of labour' (or what Schwarz (1990) calls the 'engineering of childbirth') became the central philosophy (O'Driscoll and Meagher 1980) underpinning the obstetric or medical model of pregnancy. Developing technologies are incorporated within these sets of practices and discourses, and institutional forms develop which both facilitate and constrain their use. The ability therefore of the medical professionals to influence and shape the development of the NHS in general, and maternity services in particular, is related to the powerful effects of medico-scientific discourse and the material conditions of the time. The details of these developments are chronicled elsewhere (Peretz 1990; Oakley 1986). Women's bodies have, according to Foucault, been constructed as a particular problem and in his *History of Sexuality* (1979, 1985, 1990) female sexuality was seen as in need of control and regulation. I shall examine this in more detail in Chapter 6 but it is important to note here the connections with the perceived need to control and manage pregnancy. This is an extension of the way in which women and their bodies have been problematized.

A safer place?

From the eighteenth century the obstetrician was hospital-based and the voluntary hospitals provided a good supply of women patients for them to study and treat. There were advantages to the women that used them, since they had free treatment, food and rest, but also clear benefits to the obstetricians who were able to develop teaching centres and extend their knowledge (Lewis 1980; Tew 1992, 1995). It is not known how many women nationally gave birth in institutions prior to the First World War, and the availability of maternity beds prior to 1948 is uncertain (Oakley 1986). But until the 1920s most women gave birth at home, attended by their midwife or GP (Lewis 1980; Oakley 1986; Tew 1992, 1995; Leap and Hunter 1993; Bryar 1995). A minority of women gave birth in a private nursing home or local hospital and others in workhouses and Poor Law infirmaries.

The number of hospital births was increasing (54 per cent in 1946 according to Tew 1992: 62) and the beginning of the new NHS, when maternity care became free to all, increased access to maternity beds. At that time it was believed that a hospital was the safest place to give birth. This view informed maternity policy. Changes in the funding arrangements for maternity care and payments to GPs affected the incentives for them to remain primary carers of pregnant women (Tew 1992). So, a combination of factors contributed to the rise in hospital births. The numbers of women giving birth at home reduced dramatically, commensurate with a massive rise in the numbers of hospital births. Hunt and Symonds (1995) report that in England and Wales 33.2 per cent of all births were home births in 1960 – by 1992 this figure had fallen to 1.125 per cent.

The idea that a hospital is the safest place for birth has since been hotly disputed (Campbell and McFarlane 1990, 1994; Tew 1995). In 1993 the Department of Health, following the Winterton Report (House of Commons Select Committee 1992), acknowledged this, recognizing that encouraging all women to give birth in hospital could not be justified on grounds of safety. While advocating that safety should continue to be an important consideration, they stated:

> The issue of safety, however, used as an overriding principle, may become an excuse for unnecessary interventions and technological surveillance which detract from the experience of the mother. It has to be acknowledged that some of the interventions of recent years, for example electronic fetal heart monitoring, have gained acceptance because of the assumption that they would increase the likelihood of a safe outcome. It is important that benefits are proven rather than assumed.
>
> (Department of Health 1993: 9)

Safety, it seems, has been used as a blanket justification for all kinds of interventions that are not proven to be beneficial. Ten years earlier, Oakley (1986, originally published in 1984) gave examples of hormonal treatments and mechanical devices being used for treating pre-term spontaneous abortion that were untested and unproven. Even in the absence of evidence of efficacy she says these treatments continued to be used. What was markedly different about the Department of Health's approach in 1993 was that safety was not to be seen as an 'absolute concept' but 'part of the greater picture of encompassing all aspects of health and well-being' (1993: 10).

Debates about safety and the place of birth have focused on the epidemiological evidence, the figures for maternal mortality and morbidity, and perinatal deaths of infants. In her book, Marjorie Tew (1995: 268) argues that: 'The correlations which obstetricians and others claim between increasing medical care, or specific obstetric interventions, and decreasing mortality are quickly shown to be spurious. They all fall at the first hurdle, so that further analysis is never necessary'. The common mistake that she highlights is for an association between two conditions to be taken as indicating causality. Correlations are shown to be spurious when tested to see whether there is a statistically significant relationship. In the case of falling mortality rates and medical interventions there is no such statistically significant relationship. Controversially, Tew exposed the 'lapse in logic' of earlier researchers such as the Scottish obstetrician who identified poverty and malnutrition as the most important causes of mortality but then concluded that hospital confinement would result in fewer deaths (Tew 1995: 317). She concludes that: 'by 1958 the obstetric profession, despite its much publicized conduct of self-audit, as in its Confidential Enquiries into Maternal Deaths, had already become totally impervious to evidence which discredited the success of its practices and its philosophy' (p. 325). Tew gives repeated examples of how 'unwelcome facts' were covered up.

In her discussion of *Changing Childbirth* (Department of Health 1993) Tew deplores the Expert Maternity Group's failure to support the view that non-hospital births are safer. Instead, though drawing attention to the long-standing dispute about the place of birth, 'no convincing strategy was proposed for removing the intellectual confusion and professional bias in which medical minds have become steeped after decades of unremitting brain washing' (Tew 1995: 231). She suggests that the Group perpetuated the idea that earlier debates were supported by evidence favouring the hospital as a safe place for birth, when this was not the case. Tew's criticisms culminate with the observation that obstetric intervention has been premised on the wrongly held belief that physical science provides sufficient insight into the reproductive process. However, in pointing out that 'the physical aspect of reproduction is inextricably involved with its emotional and social aspects' (Tew 1995: 378) she argues, in my view illogically, for greater attention to endocrinology – another branch of physical science! She also wants a midwifery service that relocates women in an environment that is away from obstetric intervention. The irony of Tew's analysis and criticisms of obstetrics and maternity care is that while claiming to operate within the realms of science, according to her, obstetricians *have not been scientific enough* (Tew 1995: 378). In her view they have not been rigorous enough in the application of scientific methods of investigation or interpretation of findings. In disregarding and misrepresenting the findings of scientific evidence they put self-interest and their own status as their top priority.

Socio-economic factors affecting pregnancy

Interpretation of data on the reduction of both mortality and morbidity statistics raises important theoretical and methodological issues about the factors which have contributed to improvements in maternal health. Some argue that this evidence supports developments in obstetrics and shows the efficacy of antenatal care. It is also taken as a basis for arguing that the active management of labour is justified. Others attribute these outcomes to wider changes in the material circumstances of women, and social processes. General improvements – for example, in the standard of living for the majority of mothers – have impacted on these statistics and it remains the case that the most significant factor affecting the outcome of pregnancy is the health of the mother. Variations in maternal and child health continue to be linked to poverty and class. Poverty and class both have a significant influence on the outcome of pregnancy (Whitehead 1988; Doyal 1995; Symonds and Hunt 1996).

The Winterton Report did address directly the link between poverty and pregnancy outcome and took evidence from the Department of Social Security about the levels of income support for pregnant women. Referring to debate about how far a woman's lifestyle affects her health, this committee did not support the view that pregnant women's or mothers' behaviour was the sole cause of unhealthy babies and infants. They challenged the assumptions of a simple 'lifestyle' approach to health. For example, women on low incomes may not be able to afford good quality food and could not therefore be blamed for having a poor diet. Other factors therefore needed to be taken into account, especially the effects of **material deprivation**. They concluded that the Department of Social Security was not in a position to 'comment with authority' (House of Commons Select Committee 1992: para. 133) on this since they could not provide research evidence on the matter. They made a number of recommendations for action on this issue including eligibility of young pregnant women (16–24 years) for income support, a review of special needs of families with multiple births, statutory maternity pay and family credit. Symonds and Hunt note that although the Winterton Report briefly mentioned the links between maternal health and poverty and the effects of diet and housing, 'this was not taken up by the Expert Maternity Group' (1996: 52). However, the Group themselves said 'because of its remit, it would be unable to address issues such as nutrition and socio-economic factors which can influence the outcome of pregnancy and childbirth' (Department of Health 1993: 2). The failure of the Department of Health to address the socio-economic factors affecting maternal and child health in *Changing Childbirth* is a significant limitation and indicates the political sensitivity of this issue. It also points to predictable limitations on the impact of the reforms they propose, as I shall discuss below.

Social support

In her study, *Social Support and Motherhood* (see Box 2.4) Oakley examines the connection between the social conditions of mothers and the biological

---

Box 2.4 A summary of the results of the social support and motherhood study (Oakley 1992)

- Results showed that social support for the intervention group had a positive effect on their physical health and health care use.
- Social support was relatively more helpful to those women with the most social and/or medical problems, but 'it did not help them enough to give a result which was statistically significant in terms of birthweight' (Oakley 1992: 315), even though 'results showed that babies of the intervention group had a mean birthweight 38g higher than those in the control group' (Oakley 1994: 31).
- While there was evidence that social support improved aspects of health 'the hurdles preventing the translation of this into quantative "health" effects are huge' (Oakley 1992: 316).
- Oakley concluded that providing sympathetic, listening support through continuity of care 'is a more effective way to promote pregnant women's health and that of their babies than most of the medical interventions carried out in the name of antenatal "care"' (Oakley 1992: 327).
- She says that support is best provided by other women – i.e. midwives, and that antenatal care is best at home.
- The short-term effects of social support cannot undo the health damaging effects of poverty and Oakley is anxious that such findings should not divert attention away from those health damaging effects.

---

outcomes of pregnancy. Low birth weight of a newborn baby has for some time been linked to poverty, and two thirds of low birth weight babies are born to working-class women (Oakley 1992: 13). However, according to Oakley, policy makers consistently define the problem in biological rather than social terms. Consequently she argues that policy has been directed towards the medical needs of women and has perpetuated a biomedical definition of health.

The complexity of the relationship between material deprivation and health cannot be underestimated. There are, as Oakley reminds us, both direct and indirect effects. Assessing the impact of social support on health is therefore also complicated precisely because it is an attempt to examine the points at which social and biological processes interconnect.

Oakley's 1992 study highlights in interesting ways a number of important issues that remain largely unresolved in maternity services:

- First is the issue about what counts as acceptable evidence of quality maternity services. This is both a methodological problem and a moral issue.
- Second is the relationship between what are frequently regarded as 'objective' criteria of biological indicators and the *experiences* of pregnant women. This is why much of the focus of Oakley's book is on the

construction of knowledge and a discussion of ways of knowing and understanding.

- Third, these debates are mapped onto the professional conflicts and arguments about the best place to give birth and do not examine critically the role of midwives in this process. Oakley tells us that her study was criticized for a number of reasons, and three of these, which are relevant to these issues, are discussed below.

Oakley discusses, in her (1992) book, the criticisms made of her study and the view that the experimental methods used in the study were unethical. She argues that controlled experimentation (research) is better than uncontrolled experimentation on women which, she says, characterizes clinical practice. She believes it is the lesser of two evils. The study was also criticized for not showing or explaining *how* social support works. Oakley says that it works because women acquire 'a heightened assertiveness' and are able to secure the help they feel they need and the most appropriate care. This argument is premised on the belief that women know what they need, and that what they feel they need is appropriate. This is somewhat tautological and does not attend to the ways in which women's needs are socially produced. Finally, in the study midwives provided the support, and they are professionals. Therefore some critics said that the study, if it showed anything, showed the benefits of professional support. Oakley, though clearly aware of the professional interests of obstetricians does not extend this to an analysis of the midwifery profession and rather glosses over the distinction between professional and non-professional sources of support. Instead, she accepts without question that there is 'a fundamental alignment' of midwives and women (Oakley 1992: 329), and I will return to this issue in Chapters 3 and 4.

A 'golden age' of childbirth

The Department of Health make the distinction between a medical and non-medical view of childbirth. However, it is important to recognize that this is not simply a case of non-medical personnel holding contrasting views. The success and domination of a medical/obstetric model has been because other social groups have supported, and reinforced, these dominant values and ideas. Midwives too have supported this model, becoming technocrats, managers of labour using interventionist and invasive techniques (Bryar 1995). Women themselves also welcomed the development of hospital-based care: 'Hospital birth can be seen as an example of the egalitarian and modernising ethos of the years that followed, when home birth and midwives seemed to belong to a Victorian past and were connected with memories of poverty and deprivation' (Hunt and Symonds 1995: 15).

Hospitals in the 1950s were generally seen as heralding a new and modern approach to childbirth. However, according to Hunt and Symonds they were designed for working-class women who were deferential and compliant, who would submit themselves to an assembly-line production process. But middle-class women also used these services and, during the 1970s, in the context of broader political movements, including feminism, there were growing criticisms and discontent. In Hunt and Symonds' view, midwives too reacted against hospitalization. The extent of these criticisms and their origins is a matter of debate. The National Childbirth Trust was set up in 1957 (Kitzinger 1990) but many other pressure groups are seen as originating in the feminist movement and the organization of not just middle-class women, but also working-class women (Durward and Evans 1990; Lewis 1990). The position of midwives has continued to be an ambivalent one as I shall discuss below.

Mounting criticism in the 1970s against hospital births and medicalization often appeared to hark back to a 'golden age of childbirth'. In 1977 MacIntyre was sceptical of this, saying that there was a tendency

> to suggest that childbirth was a safe, non-alienating, and beautiful experience until the advent of male medical control over the process made it into a dangerous and alienating experience. (For the villain of this history is often seen to be the male dominated medical profession which appropriated childbirth from the midwives.) The imbalance in this argument, as it is frequently presented, is that no evidence is supplied about what childbirth was like before or what it is like in primitive societies.
>
> (MacIntyre 1977: 18)

MacIntyre argued against the idea that the features of giving birth in hospital are unique to this setting, instead pointing out that in other settings similar rules and practices exist. The labouring woman is frequently restrained, or isolated and instructed by her attendants to behave in prescribed ways. Her argument was that 'the idea that human intervention in a natural physiological event is a new phenomenon' is challenged by anthropological evidence (MacIntyre 1977: 20). Moreover the assumption that normal childbirth was inherently safe is disputable. While not seeking necessarily to defend obstetric intervention, or to suggest that such an approach is without problems, MacIntyre's discussion highlights a tendency in some criticisms of medical management of labour to reconstruct the past as a golden age of childbirth (see also Leap and Hunter 1993; Bryar 1995). It raises at least two sets of interesting questions, first about what is 'normal childbirth' and second about the extent to which a return to home birth in the 1990s could radically alter the experiences of women giving birth.

Lesley Doyal warns of the dangers of underestimating the benefits of medical care:

> As many commentators have pointed out, the social context of childbirth in third world countries is often – but by no means always – a supportive one (Jordan 1983, Kitzinger 1989). The presence of loved ones, the care of a midwife and the reassurance of familiar surroundings can be of great value at what may be a time of anxiety and pain. Indeed . . . it is precisely this intimacy and solidarity that many women in developed countries feel they have lost as a result of the institutionalisation of childbirth. However moral support is not enough

when things go wrong, and some traditional practices can be dangerous. Thus all women need access to safe and effective medical care.
                                                          (Doyal 1995: 128)

Is it then that the criticisms of the past 20 years in the UK and USA are
possible only within the safer environment of a relatively affluent society
that has medical care? Some argue, notably obstetricians (Royal College of
Obstetricians and Gynaecologists 1992) that there is a danger of throwing
out the baby with the bath water, that a cry for a return to home birth
fails to recognize the benefits obstetric care have brought.

A midwifery model

In more recent midwifery literature and some feminist criticisms of the
medical model there is a view put forward that midwives are 'guardians of
the normal' (Flint 1986; Kitzinger 1988; Kitzinger *et al.* 1990; Oakley and
Houd 1990; Downe 1991). In the next chapter I shall examine how this
idea helps midwives to assert a professional identity that is distinct from
doctors, but here I want to examine the midwifery model of childbirth
which is frequently invoked by such claims.

The traditional knowledge of the midwife is seen as embedded in the
past. A past where traditional beliefs of women were regarded as 'old
wives' tales' (Dalmiya and Alcoff 1993; Leap and Hunter 1993). In a
discussion of how a hierarchy of knowledge confines certain types of
knowledge to the fringes, Dalmiya and Alcoff argue that midwives'
knowledge is epistemologically justified. Their point is that a distinction
between **propositional knowledge** (knowing that), practical skills
(knowing how) and **experiential knowledge** (being a woman) need
not necessarily imply that one type of knowledge is superior to another.
They aim to show that on epistemological grounds there is a strong case
for recognizing and valuing traditional midwives' knowledge which is
practical and based on the experience of both attending births and of
being a woman.

The history of obstetrics, is, according to Dalmiya and Alcoff (1993:
223), 'a triumph of propositional knowledge over practical knowledge'.
They argue that in certain respects midwives' knowledge was the same as
obstetrics, built up and acquired by a community of expert practitioners.
The essential difference was that it was not systematically written down
or codified. It was an oral, practical and experiential knowledge and therefore only had the status of 'old wives' tales' or traditional beliefs. 'Epistemic
discrimination' then, was based on a charge that midwives were ignorant
because they were illiterate. The significance of this is, as Dalmiya and
Alcoff point out, that practical knowledge could not be written down and
hence midwives' skills could not be reduced to propositional knowledge –
a series of rules and codes. The idea that skill is tacit or that there is an 'art
of midwifery', which is distinct from theoretical knowledge, is an important one for current debates about midwifery education (see Chapter 3).
Dalmiya and Alcoff's point is that 'the fact that midwives do not have
ordinary *propositional knowledge* does not, by itself, lead to the conclusion

Table 2.1 Midwifery and obstetrics: conceptual domains

Midwife	Obstetrician
Women	Men
Health	Disease
Normality	Abnormality
Art	Science
Social	Medical
Subjective	Objective
Experience	Knowledge
Observation	Intervention
Practice	Theory
Emotion	Reason
Intuition	Intellect
Nature	Culture
Feminine	Masculine
Community	Institution
Family	Work
Private	Public
Care	Control
Soft	Hard

Source: Oakley (1989).

that they do not have *knowledge* at all' (1993: 226). Moreover midwives, as women, have 'gender specific experiential knowledge', (1993: 228) knowledge of being a woman. The history of midwifery may then be seen as an example of how both kinds of knowledge have been discredited as not knowledge at all, since they cannot be codified. The epistemological argument against such discrimination, put forward by Dalmiya and Alcoff, is that both practical and experiential knowledge have a cognitive status and are epistemic states; that restricting what counts as knowledge to only propositional knowledge is unjustified and philosophically inadequate.

Katz Rothman (1982), Oakley (1989) and others set up an opposition between the obstetric and midwifery model of childbirth. According to Oakley, 'love' characterizes the midwife's role in childbirth and she maps a dualistic and dichotomous world where the domain of the midwife, in contrast to the obstetrician, is love, emotion, nature, normality, experience, intuition and art (see Table 2.1).

Such a dichotomy is, as Oakley recognizes, problematic. However, though claiming in many ways to be attempting to overcome these dualisms, she does appear to reproduce them in her analysis. There is a frequent assumption made by commentators, including Oakley, that midwives by virtue of being women provide a qualitatively different kind of care (Bryar 1995). This is clearly not always the case, and implies that male midwives are incapable of providing satisfactory care according to certain criteria (see Chapter 4). It also ignores female obstetricians.

As I have already indicated, midwives are often complicit in ways of working that incorporate a medical model of pregnancy and childbirth. This is sometimes explained as the result of them being restricted in their practice by the organization of services (Bryar 1995) which effectively undermines their ability to act as independent practitioners or act according to divergent principles and philosophies. I shall return to the notion of 'independent practitioner' later, but what is assumed here is that there is a direct relationship between the *organization* of care and the type of care or specific practices. While there is no doubt that they are related the relationship is not a straightforward one and they are not coterminous. In principle it is possible to imagine that many of the interventions and practices of active management could be transferred to care in the home. So, for example, drug therapies, ARM or traction applied to the placenta could continue to be features of care even for a woman giving birth at home. Similarly, the notion that 'home' can be re-created in the hospital by a few soft furnishings rather misses the point (Bryar 1995). Other types of care such as using birthing pools for pain relief or delivery, which have been seen as 'alternative' to conventional obstetric practices may be incorporated into a medicalized model of care. In the example on page 34 the use of a birthing pool was subject to similar protocol and encouragement by the Department of Health to evaluate and test the use of such pools by *clinical* criteria. This points to other processes that influence the relationship between technologies of care, institutional structures and social relationships.

A midwifery model of care usually emphasizes the importance of seeing pregnancy and birth as a natural and normal process in contrast to a pathological one. It assumes that pregnant women are healthy not sick. Following from this, radical midwives in particular claim to be 'guardians of the normal'. Such a claim glosses over the ways in which 'normal' comes to be defined in the first place. It fails to examine the ways in which 'normality' is historically, socially and culturally produced. Instead what tends to happen is that 'normal' pregnancies are attributed to those women that midwives are empowered to look after (UKCC 1991a, 1991b) and the women looked after by the obstetrician are regarded as 'abnormal' or 'high risk'. However, according to some writers, a pregnancy is frequently only defined as 'normal' retrospectively – that is, after the birth (Kitzinger *et al.* 1990). In other words, a normal pregnancy is defined as such by an uncomplicated birth. A second feature of this model is that the midwife assists the woman and is 'with woman' – the midwife is an attendant. This serves to underplay the expertise of the midwife or her specialist knowledge. The claim is that the woman has control, not the midwife. Yet contradictorily, as I show later, midwives are engaged in a professionalizing strategy which emphasizes their status and power in an attempt to wrest control from the obstetricians. At the same time practical skills of palpation and observation are usually valued more highly by midwives than theoretical and technical knowledge (Kent 1999) though this may be changing (Bryar 1995). Midwives frequently emphasize the emotional work of supporting and befriending the woman and suggest minimal use of instruments or technical equipment. They often support a holistic approach where the woman is seen as a whole person, a thinking, feeling human being (Katz Rothman 1982).

The notion of a midwifery model may be seen as an ideal. Midwives vary in the extent to which it is an ideal to which they aspire, or one they believe themselves to be operating. Bryar (1995) suggests that the medical model and the midwifery model (what she calls the model of pregnancy as a normal life-event) may be seen as on a continuum. Midwives may be seen as moving along this continuum and drawing on the two different models. Women also shift their thinking about childbirth according to different contexts and circumstances.

Ellen Annandale (1988) in her research looking at a birth centre in the USA discusses how 'natural' childbirth is an *accomplishment* of midwives. She describes how the relationships between midwives, women and obstetricians affected the way in which it was accomplished. First, women clients were socialized into thinking about childbirth as a 'natural' process. They were told it was instinctual and something which they themselves could control. Simultaneously the midwives took measures to standardize birth and carried out procedures that were designed to keep the women in the centre and prevent them from being transferred to the nearby obstetric unit, and did not stem from any belief that such measures were medically necessary. The desirability of carrying out ARM or castor oil massage was because it would enable the woman to have a 'natural' birth even though these things themselves could be regarded as interventions. In the same study women who had previously sought a natural birth gave up attempts to control the process themselves once they were transferred or admitted to the hospital. They then accepted a range of interventions, including medication for pain relief, simply because the new situation redefined the birth as 'high risk'. It was not that these were essential prerequisites for the safe delivery of the child; rather that the medical model became dominant.

Hunt and Symonds (1995) describe how for midwives in the unit they researched there was greater emphasis on getting the work done and a task-oriented approach to care rather than a focus on emotional work (see also Melia 1987). Rituals and stock phrases such as 'she's fully' or 'don't waste your pains' were used to talk to women in labour and care was routinized (Hunt and Symonds 1995). In describing interaction between midwives and the women in their care, Hunt and Symonds identify ways in which 'midwives systematically disempowered women at all stages in the childbirth experience' (1995: 93) (see also Kirkham 1983, 1989). Though they did observe occasions where 'midwives were kind, warm and compassionate human beings who were generally able to communicate very well with women' and there was evidence of 'good practice', their other examples show how varied practice can be (Hunt and Symonds 1995: 92). This account sits uneasily with the notion of a midwifery model of care. Hunt and Symonds explain these observations with reference to the organization of midwifery work in the hospital. Essentially, according to this analysis, the need to control and organize the work leads to certain practices and behaviour by the midwifery workforce. This functionalist analysis offers little insight into the reasons why such organizational imperatives may have arisen in the first place.

Hunt and Symonds (1995) provide a useful ethnographic description of midwifery work in *The Social Meaning of Midwifery*. The authors outline how midwives may be seen as 'the aristocracy of female labour' (p. 140) because midwifery is a skilled female occupation. In their discussion of skill as a gendered concept they suggest that midwives have been de-skilled since moving into the high-tech environment of the hospital. Simultaneously they have achieved professional status and 'a recognis-able occupational space within professional health care' (p. 142). I will return to this in Chapter 4, but what is interesting here is the belief of some midwives that traditional midwifery skills may be developed outside the high-tech obstetric unit in midwifery-led units or in the community. Midwives have acquired new skills as new technologies have come into common usage but this has been associated with their subordination as obstetric nurses assisting the obstetrician. In contrast the older, traditional skills that predate the modern era are valued because they are attributed to the midwife as an independent practitioner. The concept of skill there-fore is closely tied to the extent of control the midwife has over her own work.

Hunt and Symonds oversimplify the relations between knowledge and power in the maternity services. They conclude that in relation to 'the key issues of control, continuity and choice were in essence issues of commun-ication' (1995: 147). They say that the availability of more information will enable women to make choices about the care they receive. While this is an important way of improving maternity care, we cannot assume that information is neutral. In addition, we need to examine the other factors that constrain women in making those choices, and the con-straints operating on midwifery practice.

Gendered knowledge

In setting up an opposition between the medical and midwifery model of pregnancy and childbirth, feminist sociologists such as Oakley, Katz Rothman and myself are drawing on a large body of feminist literature that has developed a critique of scientific and medical practice. It is fre-quently argued that medicine is a **patriarchal** discourse, that the lan-guage and practice of medical science systematically oppresses women. Certainly there is considerable evidence to support such a view. Women are under-represented in the management of the NHS, at the policy mak-ing level and in senior positions in medicine. Women are frequently excluded in the setting of research agendas and as participants in health research (Doyal 1994, 1998). Women have been subject to the increased effects of medicalization in certain areas of their lives (notably reproduc-tion) and have also been marginalized. In the area of mental health too, diagnosis and treatment has been developed along divisions of gender (Busfield 1996). However, the direction of these developments and the ways they have affected groups of women and individuals are complex. As Doyal (1994: 146) says there is a danger of seeing accounts of medicalization as 'over-determined in their negative assessment of the benefits some medical techniques can offer women, in their exaggeration of the power of individual doctors and in their assumptions of the universality of unre-mitting sexism among all practitioners'. Doyal argues that there is also an underlying conspiracy model of 'nasty' doctors. She concludes that a more interactive understanding of doctor-patient relations and a focus on impact or outcomes rather than intentions is needed.

There are a number of issues which Doyal draws attention to here. First, women are not cultural dopes and have been active in contributing to their own oppression by the acceptance and use of medical definitions of pregnancy and childbirth, health and illness. But they have also been active in opposing and resisting medical practices through consumer groups such as the National Childbirth Trust and the Association for Improvements to Maternity Services (Durward and Evans 1990; Kitzinger 1990), and in questioning the care they receive. Solidarity has been important in opposing certain developments. Second, not all women are the same; increased attention in feminist theory to diversity and difference argues that women are not a homogenous group. With respect to health services, divisions of class, race and ethnicity (Phoenix 1990), disability and sexuality (Wilton 1997) have affected the care that women have received. Third, doctors have been treated as a homogenous group, an army of men that has conspired to oppress women. This is not straightforwardly the case; individual doctors may well be sympathetic and helpful to women's needs (Savage 1988; 1990). However, to suggest that the intentions of individual doctors have been the focus of criticisms, psychologizes and individualizes the problem. Though it seems quite appropriate to suggest that a focus of empirical enquiry should be the actions of doctors, Doyal (1994) does not explore how such actions are constituted as either oppressive or liberating. She also misses the significance of her own suggestion that an interactionist perspective is needed. We need to distinguish between the actions of individual practitioners and the effects of medical discourse.

Discourse theory of knowledge

Part of the difficulty is that when we do focus on health services and medical practices there is a tendency to neglect the relationship between *knowledge* and practice. Practice, or action, is embedded in language and a discourse theory of knowledge emphasizes this. It follows therefore that in the field of maternity services, the interactional aspects of day-to-day maternity care which produce, and are structured by, the relationships between women and their carers are very significant. It is not, as Hunt and Symonds (1995) suggest, simply that information needs to be shared, though they are right to point out that this is important. In addition, we need to understand how 'information' becomes structured in certain ways. This means that *communication is important* because it constitutes these relationships and reproduces them. However, at the same time communication is frequently constrained and inequalities always remain which may distort it. So the actions of doctors and midwives, embedded in the language they use to talk about what they do, may simultaneously include and exclude women, liberate and oppress them. To explain this more fully let us take as an example the case study shown in Box 2.5.

Box 2.5 A case study – using a birthing pool

In 1997, four years after *Changing Childbirth* (Department of Health 1993) a woman I know was soon to give birth when the hospital where she had booked for a delivery announced that if she wanted to use the birthing pool she had to sign an agreement to take part in a research project. She was told this would involve certain tests being carried out, including electronic foetal monitoring during the labour. She questioned this policy and sought advice from the supervisor of midwives who upheld the position. The woman asked for a copy of the research protocol. She then asked my advice. I obtained for her a letter from the chair of the hospital medical research ethics committee which advised that 'the act of using the birthing pool is an experiment' (MaClean 1997, personal communication). I also obtained verbal comments from members of AIMS (Association for Improvements to Maternity Services) on the situation who, while wanting to support the woman in her own choice of care, were strongly critical of the hospital and its policies. They were critical of a government policy that supported women-centred care but not midwifery-led services. Sharing these comments with the woman and leaving her to make up her own mind about what to do next, I reflected on what had happened.

In the case study, what lay at the centre of the woman's dilemma about whether to go ahead and use the birthing pool was that it was part of an experiment. (The woman had already had experience herself of using a birthing pool at a different hospital for the birth of her first child.) By constructing 'act of using the birthing pool' in this way the ethics committee invoked a powerful medico-scientific discourse to position the woman as an experimental subject and as doing something (that is, giving birth in water) which was a legitimate focus of scientific inquiry. The issue of consent was that by appearing to give a 'choice' about whether or not she used the pool, she also 'chose' to take part in the research. Of course there were 'alternatives', other options, as the members of AIMS pointed out. She could go somewhere else, she could hire her own pool (if she could afford it) or have her baby at home. But whatever she did she was both caught in and resisting the discourses around pregnancy and childbirth which enable such 'choices' to be specified as options in the first place. The actions and talk of the hospital midwives and doctors defined the 'alternatives'. If the woman sought to challenge the hospital further, she would be drawn into the contrasting discourses and practices of birth activists, who seek to improve and change the maternity services and frequently adopt an oppositional position to the dominant medical one. But, by virtue of their opposition, they reproduce, and to some degree perpetuate, the very practices they seek to oppose. This is the paradox that a Foucauldian analysis of knowledge and power highlights.

Experiential knowledge

Many feminist critiques of science have drawn attention to the ways in which the experience of women is neglected and marginalized. (In Chapter 7 I examine this with reference to the development of new reproductive technologies.) There is a long-standing debate within the philosophy of social sciences about the relationship between theoretical, practical and experiential knowledge already referred to above. In feminist theory the extent to which *experience* provides the basis of valid knowledge has been of particular concern. To summarize these debates briefly, the argument centres around the relationship between language and experience. For some writers such as Stanley and Wise (1993) 'Being' is foundational, and by virtue of being women, we have a unique position in the world from which to understand and know (things). Harding (1986, 1991) also argues for a standpoint theory of knowledge and believes that by recognizing that we are all positioned in the world in certain ways, and using our knowledge of that position, we can become more objective about the world. However, Scott (1992) says that experience is discursively mediated; that we cannot use experience to explain the world but rather it is experience itself which needs to be explained. The debate has been frequently framed as an opposition between **essentialism/foundationalism** on the one hand and **constructionism** on the other, but a closer reading of these writers' work often suggests that the differences between them are not always as significant as first appears (see Chapters 6 and 7).

Stanley and Wise (1993), though criticized for their foundationalism, acknowledged that experience is discursively mediated, organized and structured by language and power. It seems that the widest area of disagreement is the direction of influence one upon the other. Does experience lead to certain kinds of knowledge or do certain kinds of knowledge shape and influence our experience of a situation? It seems to me that the implications of what is said for feminist praxis is that we need to see each acting upon the other. So in the example above (see Box 2.5), the experience of having already given birth in a birthing pool at another hospital constructed the woman's view and expectations for the second birth. However, the knowledge she now has about the way in which other health professionals talk about, view and act with regard to the birthing pool shaped her experience of this birth. All these factors interact. The bodily experience of giving birth is constructed at the point where these factors connect (see Figure 2.1).

The difficulty with talking about pregnancy and childbirth from the point of view of a medical or midwifery model is that neither are, in

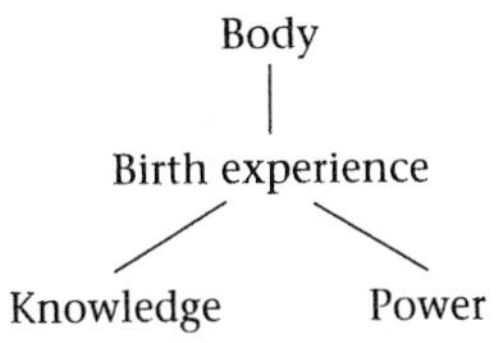

Figure 2.1 Constructing experience

practice or daily use, entirely distinct from each other. They overlap and are used by different groups including midwives, doctors and women. There have also been some changes in how they are used. Increasingly, biomedical definitions of health have been extended to include social and psychological aspects. While this may be interpreted as a modification, or dilution of exclusively biological and clinical indicators, it may also be seen as an extension of medicine (and nursing, see Porter 1998) to new areas of social control. Social medicine incorporates social aspects within a medical model rather than adopting a social model of medicine. Moreover, even if social factors are recognized as influencing maternal and child health, this does not necessarily lead to measures targeted to improve the position of disadvantaged groups (for example poor pregnant women), as already indicated.

In relation to midwifery there is a contradictory set of tendencies. There is often an emphasis on practical skills and traditional knowledge which may arguably be seen as pre-scientific or pre-modern since it looks backwards to the 'wise woman' of the past (Alcoff and Potter 1993). At the same time midwives are actively engaged in strategies for improving their professional status which, as we shall see in the next chapter, appear to rely on developing greater theoretical competences (Kent *et al.* 1994; Bryar 1995; Kent 1995). In many situations this includes their reskilling, using modern technologies (Hunt and Symonds 1995). There has been a strong argument put forward to give voice to women's own experiences of pregnancy and childbirth as part of an emancipatory project. This emancipatory discourse runs through much of the midwifery literature, especially among radical midwives (Kent 1995, forthcoming). By aligning themselves 'with women' midwives claim to act in their interests, to be women working with women. Such a claim has not been entirely accepted by the Department of Health (1993) or the House of Commons Select Committee (1992). They recognized that many women feel that midwives are best placed to provide their care, and therefore should be able to choose to be cared for by a midwife. But the Committee and the Expert Maternity Group did not consider that midwives either have a *right* to care for women, or that changes in childbirth should be directed to giving greater control to any one professional group. *Changing Childbirth* was permissive in that it acknowledged that midwives *may* be the lead professionals in a woman's care but it did not advocate a midwife-led service. The extent of changes likely to be implemented is a contentious issue.

Women know best – the future of maternity services

I will discuss more fully women's experiences of pregnancy later in the book but the principle that women know best is of concern here. The Department of Health (1993) identified three key principles of good maternity care:

● The woman is the focus of care, in control of what is happening to her and making decisions about care, based on her needs, in consultation with health professionals.

- Maternity services should be accessible and based primarily in the community.
- Women should be involved in monitoring and planning effective and efficient services.

Both purchasers and providers of maternity services were expected to review services and consider a strategy for implementing changes in the light of the recommendations made in *Changing Childbirth* (Department of Health 1993). Changes proposed were directed towards a more women-centred service, where women could carry their own notes, have a greater say in their care and a wider choice of services. Each woman would have a named midwife from whom she could obtain advice. Women could choose to book their care with a midwife who could act as a 'lead professional' throughout the pregnancy and birth. Home birth should be a real option for women, partnerships between GPs and midwives were to be encouraged and GP training reviewed. Midwives should make full use of their skills while the obstetrician's role is to care for women with complicated pregnancies, but they should also be available to other women. Consumer representation at the local level should include diverse groups. Accessible and unbiased information should be made available along with a monitoring of services to ensure that disadvantaged women take those services up. Clinical audit, evidence-based practice and a more community oriented service should be established.

The concept of a women-centred service is premised on the view that a woman is capable of making decisions about the care she receives. In certain respects this suggests a break with the past. Historically in the UK the provision of welfare services has been patterned by the notion of universal rights and citizenship. In political theory and philosophy, this rights-based model of social justice has been debated. From a feminist perspective, the notion of universal rights renders the rights of women invisible. Women as subjects, undifferentiated from men, have been marginalized in a welfare system that assumes a woman is dependent on a man and where her entitlement to services has been determined by her relationship to a man (see Chapter 5). The development of maternity services grew from an extension of universal rights for women. In this regard it was a significant gain and benefit to women's health. However, the idea that rights to welfare include anything other than access to services, the form and kind of which were determined by the health professionals and technocrats who manage them (what Klein 1983 referred to as paternalism), was not part of that earlier thinking. Significantly the proposals for change may mark something of a triumph for activists who have campaigned for greater rights for women, and improvements to maternity services (for example AIMS). However, the extent to which this represents a moral and political victory is not clear. Has much changed? This question may be considered in at least three ways. First, what changes (if any) have occurred in the kind of services available? Second, has there been a radical rethinking of the way in which pregnancy and childbirth is now viewed – a paradigm shift or epistemological challenge to medicine (or midwifery)? Third, have women secured bodily autonomy and integrity in the new maternity services?

Box 2.6 Is childbirth really changing?

In an article published by the National Childbirth Trust the following findings were reported on a study carried out in 1994 (Gready et al. 1995). The study, which included 850 women in Essex, found that 31 per cent had previously met one of the midwives who cared for them in labour and 47 per cent would like to get to know their doctor or midwife better, but over half said they didn't want to know them any better. Few women had been given a choice about where to give birth. Only 13 per cent were offered a home birth and some had fought to have a home birth. There was also limited choice about antenatal care. Over half the women wanted more information.

The Audit Commission's study of maternity services discussed by Robinson was reported to show that women frequently do not have a choice in where they go for antenatal care, whether their labour is induced or augmented. Only half of the 3500 women surveyed had 'felt they definitely had a say as to whether to have a scan and 60 per cent in whether they had screening tests' (Robinson 1997: 62). Other findings indicated widespread variation in care and continuing dispute about what constitutes appropriate care especially for some groups of women.

Changes in service provision

The implementation team set up in 1994 to promote change in maternity services report on exciting developments and projects supported by monies set aside to take forward the recommendations of the Department of Health (Jackson 1995). Examples of good practice were to be extended through networking and the sharing of information. Others however suggest that there has been 'patchy progress' (Waters 1996) (see Box 2.6).

Changes in midwifery practice

In the midwifery press there has been concern about the increased accountability of midwives in a service where they are expected to have greater autonomy and act as lead professionals (Symon 1995). Clinical accountability in midwife-led units and a community-based service are seen as of considerable importance and linked to this is the need for professional indemnity insurance to protect midwives from liability suits. At the same time, the insurance cover available to independent midwives working outside the NHS has become more difficult to secure (Flint 1997; Lewis 1997). The sphere of practice for the midwife, linked to the concept of 'normality', is expected to widen and the boundaries of 'normal' to be redefined (Symon 1995). The working conditions and pay for midwives have been criticized as not reflecting their new responsibilities and increased workload. Controversially no transfer of resources to the community to facilitate change was reported (Walsh and Crompton 1997; Waters 1996).

Fears have been expressed that a campaign to promote consumer awareness was premature because changes had not been implemented (Waters 1996).

Wide variation in what constitutes midwife-led care is evident and guidelines for this kind of service are still being developed, since the criteria used to determine whether women may opt for midwifery care rather than obstetric care have not been universally agreed (Walsh and Crompton 1997). Walsh and Crompton's discussion about the ways in which women are referred between midwives and obstetricians reveals a continuing concern about who 'captures' the woman. Moreover, the increased tendency in some midwifery units for midwives to augment (speed up) labour and carry out ventouse/forceps deliveries throws into dispute further the distinction between midwifery and obstetric care, or any concept of a normal delivery as a natural one. Other debates about the skills a midwife needs in order to practise in the community include the setting up of intravenous infusions and their role in obstetric emergencies (Walton and Hamilton 1995: 66). Support for 'evidence-based midwifery practice' is seen as raising the 'important question about what constitutes evidence' and as creating a career structure for midwife researchers (Walsh and Crompton 1997: 116). It also raises questions about 'What is midwifery?' Walton and Hamilton (1995) and Sleep (1995) identify other areas for research in midwifery and where changes in practice might be implemented in the light of *Changing Childbirth* (Department of Health 1993).

Rights and choices

The recognition of a woman's right to choose where she gives birth and to have a greater say in the type of care she receives invokes a set of ideas about the relationship between rights and choices. It also adopts a model of democracy where the woman, as a consumer of maternity services, is expected to be able to exercise her rights and make choices. Closer attention to the premises that underlie such a view points to a number of difficulties which remain for women. On the issue of choice it was noted in 1993 that women are frequently denied real choice and 'more research, especially in the form of large-scale studies, is needed to expand knowledge of the particular choices that are important to women' (Department of Health 1993: 98). Women were recognized as not being a homogenous group. Differences were considered important and therefore a need for a flexible service was identified. Clearly some women have more choice than others, with greater control over their lives and what happens to them when they become pregnant. Home birth is more likely to be an option for women who have decent housing. Renting a birthing pool will only be an option to those who can afford it. The increase in the number of Caesarean deliveries and the resulting negative effects have been explored in the literature (Oakley and Richards 1990). Reports that women are being submitted to surgery for Caesarean section against their own wishes suggest that a woman's right to choose her care is being violated. The justification for court orders being given in these cases is premised on the belief that women in labour are incapable of making decisions and are temporarily insane. Women are not even represented in court hearings when their case is discussed (Kenny 1996). This appears to fly in the face of claims that a women-centred service is being developed. Conversely, other women are claiming the right to choose to have a Caesarean section as a way of exercising greater control and planning the time of their delivery (Robinson 1998). Just what a woman-centred service should look like is a complex issue.

Although the Department of Health advocate greater choice and a wider range of services they also acknowledge that:

> there are factors beyond the scope of the maternity services, such as low incomes, poor housing and inadequate nuturition, that can have a decisive influence on a woman's experience by decreasing choice, restricting access to services and increasing risks to her and her baby. While the NHS needs to provide services which mitigate the effect of these disadvantages, there are obvious limits as to what can be done by health care alone.
>
> (Department of Health 1993: 98)

Clearly there are limits to the extent to which greater choice for women can be achieved. Inequalities will remain between women but also between women and health professionals.

There is an explicit attempt to have lay or consumer representatives on the statutory maternity liaison committees. However, it is likely that even here, representatives from marginal groups of women will face difficulties in becoming members of such a body. This is not to imply that representation is not useful, but the terms and conditions under which a consumer representative may act within such a group will continue to be constrained by wider social and political processes. Women, seen as consumers, are constrained by a discourse of the market place.

There are a number of difficulties with the very idea of pregnant women as consumers. It is contentious how far a liberal discourse of rights and choices is appropriate for discussing maternity services for the same reasons that it is problematic when discussing the new reproductive technologies (see Chapter 7). The *Patients' Charter*, which introduces the idea of a named midwife for each pregnant woman provides a framework for extending choice but its force seems limited.

A continuing problem is how women may make professionals *accountable* for their practice, especially at a time when they are relatively dependent on those same professionals for access to their services. Consumer bodies such as the National Childbirth Trust, while offering support for home birth, do not take up the cases of individual women to argue for particular kinds of care. In the example given in Box 2.5 (see page 34) members of AIMS did volunteer to attend the antenatal clinic with the woman wanting to use the birthing pool, but even this could potentially have led to a decrease in her control over what then happened. She remained fearful of the effects of alienating or upsetting the professionals who cared for her.

Challenging medicine?

This chapter aimed to look at competing approaches to pregnancy and childbirth, to examine the question 'Who knows best?' I have sought to show how doctors, midwives and women may be seen as having differing ways of knowing. I suggested that midwives and doctors are frequently represented as in opposition to each other. Such opposition commonly seeks to advance the political project of one or other group. So for example, midwives who oppose medical management of pregnancy and childbirth constitute the medical profession as villains, who exploit women and deskill midwives in order to assert their authority as experts. Midwives align themselves with women since women often prefer a midwife to care for them. In arguing for changes in childbirth, midwives and other consumer groups have argued for a midwife-led service. This has not been proposed by the Department of Health though it appears that there is likely to be an increase in midwife-led units and a shift to community-based services. However, in the absence of a transfer of resources to facilitate this, it is hard to assess what in the longer term a reformed maternity service will look like.

At the same time therefore it is possible to argue that little has changed, that there has not been a fundamental shift in power from obstetricians to midwives. In so far as midwives pay and working conditions remain the same there is little to suggest that midwives will enjoy the status and position of obstetricians. More importantly for this analysis, it seems that the obstetric profession remains intact. The response of the Royal College of Obstetricians and Gynaecologists (1992) to the Winterton Report (House of Commons Select Committee, 1992) was defiant and as Tew (1995) argued, the Expert Maternity Group did not substantially undermine the obstetricians' position that a hospital is safe, despite evidence to the contrary. Moreover, rather than midwives being able to assert traditional skills there is some indication that their practices will include techniques previously carried out by the obstetrician (for example, forceps delivery). In addition what seems to be happening in some hospitals is that 'alternative approaches' to childbirth are being incorporated within the dominant discourse and practices. So for example, the constitution of the birthing pool as part of an experiment is premised on a model of knowledge production that is within the scientific paradigm. The concept of discourse therefore is useful because rather than tying knowledge to specific subject positions we can begin to see that ideas about pregnancy and childbirth cannot easily be confined to distinct and separate groups. Midwives and women have sometimes also adopted a medicalized view of pregnancy and childbirth.

Evidence-based practice and clinical audit continue to emphasize *clinical* aspects of care as meriting attention. The social is usually added-in as a variable rather than being considered as fundamentally challenging the way in which clinical outcomes are *socially* produced. A hierarchy of knowledge remains, with the methods and techniques of scientific medicine being applied to new areas of midwifery and medical practice. Hunt and Symonds (1995) say that currently midwives, not women (or doctors), control birth in most instances. If changes increase the number of instances where midwives are the lead professionals, or teams of midwives provide continuity of carer, there seems to be a possibility of enhancing the midwives' control, but this could be at the expense of the woman. While many women do prefer the care of midwives, and midwives are often more 'woman-centred', the assumption that the interests of mid-wives and women are the same is problematic, though this is frequently taken to be the case. It remains to be seen whether a woman-centred service reverses the direction of a hierarchy of knowledge that has charac-terized maternity services and whether the experiences of women will be valued as highly as the technical or propositional knowledge of the obstetrician or professional midwife.

Conclusions

It is not at all clear that the knowledge and experience of the woman is being prioritized or valued. There is a suggestion that the professionals may not always know best but there is no fundamental challenge to their claim to knowledge. Obstetricians are still thought to know best in cases of complicated pregnancy. The named midwife concept explicitly recog-nizes that *professional* help is what may be needed, in contrast to a special friend, or mentor who is a mother herself, or even the woman's own mother. Such other sources of help and advice are not legitimated by the proposed new approach to maternity care. As a result individual women may continue to feel isolated by their experience of pregnancy, and the extent to which bodily integrity and autonomy for mothers may be achieved remains severely circumscribed (see Chapters 5 and 8). There may indeed be a proliferation of options for women, a growth in the number of birthing pools available in the hospital (or community). But there is little to suggest that a fundamental and radical change in the way in which professional knowledge of pregnancy and childbirth is prioritized has occurred or is likely to occur through reorganizing service provision. A woman-centred approach to care represents a step forward but translat-ing this into practice depends on powerful groups of health professionals being prepared to give account of their practice to women. Women are still in the position of only being able to make professionals accountable through the courts and liability action or complaints to the community health councils. This is an onerous and difficult task for anyone and especially for those women who are most often neglected by public services.

In addition a transfer of resources to women is needed to overcome the effects of poverty and material deprivation, to improve maternal and child health. Whether the NHS research and development programme in mother and child health can deliver this is an open question (Department of Health 1995). In the meantime, when midwives focus on the need to transfer resources to them, the debate about how to effect improvements continues to be framed in terms of clinical and professional imperatives. This does not assist in empowering women to take care of themselves and manage their own lives with the assistance of their elected helpers. Clearly the vision for future maternity services is a more highly trained profes-sional midwife with a greater field of competence and practice than has been seen in recent years. Changes in midwifery education discussed in the next chapter are closely linked to this vision.

Summary

- Chapter 2 has examined the development of modern maternity services and the current debate about the implementation of changes in the NHS. I have used key sociological concepts to explain these changes and have drawn on the work of theorists such as Foucault, Weber and Turner.

- The processes of secularization, scientization, rationalization and bureaucratization are seen as central to the development of modern health care systems.

- The development of scientific medical knowledge and the medicalization of pregnancy and childbirth in the nineteenth and twentieth centuries have influenced the kind of care pregnant and labouring women receive.

- Predating these developments are the traditional skills and knowledge of midwives that have been marginalized and transformed over time. I described the differences between the medical and midwifery models of pregnancy and childbirth and how conflicts between the professions have influenced recent policy decisions.

- The stated intention that maternity services are to become more woman-centred was seen as implying that women's own knowledge and experience should be more highly valued. However, I conclude that the conditions under which women are able to choose the care they wish for themselves are frequently restrictive.

- Although women may be regarded as consumers their ability to make professions accountable to them is severely limited. My analysis therefore points to the need to understand how knowledge and power are intimately connected and a sociological approach to knowledge helps us to do this.

Discussion points

- What characterizes the development of maternity care in the twentieth century?

- Outline the debate surrounding the obstetric or medical model of pregnancy and childbirth.

- What evidence is there to demonstrate links between social conditions and pregnancy outcomes?

- In what sense do midwives appear to draw on different kinds of knowledge claims to medical men?

- Is knowledge gendered?

- How far has the belief that 'women know best' shaped current policy and practice in maternity services?

Further reading

Alcoff, L. and Potter, E. (eds) (1993) *Feminist Epistemologies*. London: Routledge.

Department of Health (1993) *Changing Childbirth, Part 1: Report of the Expert Maternity Group*. London: HMSO.

Doyal, L. (1995) *What Makes Women Sick? Gender and the Political Economy of Health*. London: Macmillan.

Hunt, S. and Symonds, A. (1995) *The Social Meaning of Midwifery*. London: Macmillan.

Leap, N. and Hunter, B. (1993) *The Midwife's Tale: An Oral History from Handywoman to Professional Midwife*. London: Scarlet Press.

Oakley, A. (1992) *Social Support and Motherhood: The Natural History of a Research Project*. Oxford: Blackwell.

Porter, S. (1998) *Social Theory and Nursing Practice*. London: Macmillan.

Tew, M. (1995) *Safer Childbirth?: A Critical History of Maternity Care*, 2nd edn. London: Chapman & Hall.

Turner, B. (1992) *Regulating Bodies: Essays in Medical Sociology*. London: Routledge.

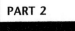

PART 2

THE PROFESSIONALS

EDUCATING THE PROFESSIONALS

Introduction

So far I have explored how competing approaches to childbirth and different ways of knowing have shaped contemporary maternity services. The
emphasis in the last chapter was on developing an understanding about
what counts as knowledge. Midwifery knowledge was seen as frequently
undervalued and the status of midwives was linked to the domination of
a scientific or medicalized view of pregnancy and childbirth. In this chapter
I shall examine how recent changes in midwifery education and developments in the midwifery curriculum may be linked to the development of

new forms of midwifery knowledge. At the same time, I suggest that by adopting a sociological perspective of these changes we can begin to see how knowledge and power are closely related. These new forms of knowledge will also affect the social relationships of midwives. The education debate, then, has been about the future of the midwifery profession and the direction which midwifery practice might take.

This chapter also introduces the concept of *identity* in order to show how midwifery knowledge *produces* a midwife. In a discussion of student midwives I shall show how identifying themselves as midwives is a central part of the education process. However, becoming a midwife is seen as a dynamic process, not simply a new uniform which the student puts on or new knowledge which the student acquires. The process of *identification* is important in creating a sense of belonging to a group. It also helps to create a distinction or boundary between those who are midwives and those who are not, to determine who may belong. This I shall argue is a key part of the way in which midwives seek to establish their professional status.

So let us turn to professional and educational issues and focus on midwifery education and training. I want to examine the development of today's professional midwife and the changes in midwifery education that have occurred. In particular I shall describe the development of pre-registration midwifery education in England since 1989 and the implications of this for the midwifery profession. My focus is England because I am drawing on research I carried out in that country between 1991 and 1993. However, the changes in UKCC (United Kingdom Central Council for Nursing, Midwifery and Health Visiting) policy have also been important in shaping midwifery education in Scotland, Wales and Northern Ireland. This chapter will give you an insight into professional politics in an education setting. A sociological analysis of policy changes enables us to consider how midwives have engaged in professionalizing strategies in order to secure occupational territory, status and power. This analysis develops on three levels which, although discussed in turn, may be seen as interconnected.

- At the *policy* level I shall show how professional power has been a central concern for midwives. It has been at the centre of attempts to gain autonomy and be self-regulating. An historical account of the transition from lay midwife to professional is the starting point for this discussion.
- At the level of the *educational institution* (the colleges of health and universities where midwifery education is now located) I argue that professional rivalries between midwives and nurses have been important in shaping the form and development of individual educational programmes. At the same time, in the context of higher education, midwives face new pressures.
- At the level of the *student* the process of becoming a midwife will be seen as a discursive process whereby students mobilize certain kinds of accounts of what it means to be a midwife. In so doing they position themselves in relation to other students, the nursing profession and midwifery colleagues.

From lay midwife to professional midwife

Historical accounts of the development of midwifery record the transition from the handywoman, wise woman or lay midwife to the professional midwife at the turn of the twentieth century. In their fascinating book, *The Midwife's Tale*, Leap and Hunter (1993) tell the stories of some of the handywomen who were called upon to attend births, lay out the dead and tend the sick. Historical and literary accounts of what these women were like include both negative images of slovenly, drunken and unclean 'old gamps', and positive ones of conscientious, clean, caring and dedicated women who were pillars of their community. It is the latter of these which emerges in Leap and Hunter's book. For poor and working-class women the lay midwife or handywoman was the preferred form of assistance, not least because her services were affordable. For the middle-class woman the option of more expensive medical care was available. According to Leap and Hunter, in the late nineteenth century 'an elite group of philanthropic women from middle-class, upper middle-class and aristocratic backgrounds spearheaded a campaign to regulate the training and practice of midwives' (1993: 2).

Their efforts led to the establishment of the first regulatory body, the Midwives Institute and the 1902 Midwives Act. (For an account of the parallel struggle for nurse registration see Rafferty 1996.) Towler and Bramall (1986) report that training for midwives had already been available in the nineteenth century when midwives were trained in the lying-in hospitals (see Versluyen 1981). They say that Florence Nightingale's vision was for well trained, intelligent and educated women to be midwives (and nurses) who would consult doctors only when necessary. The increased concern to both regulate and legitimate medical practice had implications for the control of midwifery practice as doctors and midwives competed for maternity patients.

As obstetrics became a recognized branch of medicine in the late nineteenth century, the concern was that the role of the midwife and the doctor should be carefully demarcated. Powerful medical men sought to protect their sphere of practice and their income, but though fees for childbirth were lucrative, many preferred to leave the care of labouring women to the midwife. Towler and Bramall (1986), Donnison (1977) and others have highlighted the opposition to attempts to upgrade the midwife and recognize her as a formally qualified practitioner. Eight attempts to introduce legislation failed before the 1902 Act was passed (Towler and Bramall 1986). Together with later midwives acts this legislative framework established the new professional midwife as having a statutory responsibility to attend childbirth. It became illegal for anyone else to attend a birth 'habitually or for gain, except under the direction of a doctor, unless she was certified under the Act' (Towler and Bramall 1986: 180). Midwives were certified under the Act after a formal period of training that initially was three months. Twentieth-century midwifery legislation is summarized in Box 3.1.

Box 3.1   Midwifery legislation 1902–97

1902   Midwives Act – midwives are licensed to practise; rules
         regulating practice are established

1920   Midwives Act – provision made for midwives to be appointed
         to the Central Midwife Board although numbers restricted to a
         minority of 5/14

1936   Midwives Act – local authorities required to provide a
         midwifery service

1951   Midwives Act – consolidated legislation of 1902, 1918, 1926
         and 1950

1973   NHS Act – removed responsibility for personal health services
         from local authorities to the NHS

1979   Nurses, Midwives and Health Visitors Act – established the UK
         Central Council for Nursing, Midwifery and Health Visiting
         (UKCC) and the four national boards: English, Welsh, Scottish
         and Northern Ireland

1980   European Community directives – specified the responsibilities
         of member states to ensure that midwives are able to carry out
         certain duties

1992   Nurses, Midwives and Health Visitors Act Amendment – the
         role of the national boards focused on implementation of
         standards and their composition altered; the UKCC was made
         the elected body

1997   A review of the Nurses, Midwives and Health Visitors Act –
         consultation about the future regulatory role of the UKCC and
         the national boards following the integration of health care
         professional education into higher education institutions

The role of the midwife in law

Since 1902 the role of the midwife has been legally defined and formal
rules developed to guide her practice (UKCC 1991a, 1991b). Requirements
for education and training have changed and a detailed account of the
early changes is found in Towler and Bramall (1986). Since 1916 there
have been two routes to a midwifery qualification: a 'direct entry' route
and a shortened course for those who are trained nurses. By 1981 the
length of training for the direct entrant was three years, and for the
qualified nurse, 18 months. These changes brought training in the UK
into line with European directives (EEC 1980) (see Box 3.2).

   The licensing and certification of midwives may be seen as serving a
number of purposes and having certain consequences. The introduction
of formal training requirements marked a move towards **'credentialism'**,

a strategy for professionalizing groups (Hugman 1991; Witz 1992) including nurses (Rafferty 1996). Devries (1982) suggests that there is a dual purpose to licensing midwifery practice. It is both enabling, in so far as it recognizes the value of what midwives do, and disabling in limiting the scope of their action. This view is reiterated by Oakley and Houd (1990: 24) who assert that the midwives' 'professional relationship with doctors began to be defined and codified to the midwives' increasing disadvantage with the emergence of professionalised medicine'. According to their analysis, the professionalization of midwives is closely tied to medicine and can be traced back to the 1880s (see also Donnison 1977). Through the licensing process of both medical and midwifery practitioners, '**occupational closure**' (Hugman 1991; Witz 1992) was sought. As a professional group, midwives aimed to control who could practise midwifery. However, the ability of the midwifery profession to regulate its own practice was, as Oakley and Houd (1990) identify, strictly limited.

Witz (1992: 116) also draws attention to the limits placed on midwives, arguing that 'the midwife was to enjoy discretion at the level of execution in her daily practice as an independent practitioner with her own clients, but within a sphere of competence prescribed by the medical profession and restricted to attendance on normal labour'. Witz argues that both midwives and medical men used a variety of strategies to demarcate their occupational role. Medical men in favour of midwifery registration supported a 'demarcationary strategy of de-skilling' (Witz 1992: 109) which allowed for a separate and independent practitioner midwife. Those opposed to registration (mainly general practitioners) sought to abolish the independent midwifery role and incorporate all aspects of midwifery into their own practice. But at the end of the day, the deskilling strategy prevailed. This was partly because the demand for midwifery services could not be satisfied by medical men and the poor would not be able to afford their services. Crucially, midwives could practise independently in attendance at a 'normal' labour, but the medical men maintained control over 'abnormal' labours.

According to Witz the ability of medical men to engage in such a demarcationary strategy is linked to their dominant status within patriarchal society. Interprofessional conflicts are gendered, and in contrast the midwives engaged in 'female professional projects' of **dual closure**. They made use of 'exclusionary strategies' to restrict entry into the profession and used 'credentialist and legalistic tactics' (Witz 1992: 117). But in accepting the limitations on their practice and knowledge base, the Midwives Institute adopted an 'accommodative strategy' which Witz says enabled them to maintain a degree of autonomy, albeit within strict limits. Moreover, the governing bodies set up to regulate and control midwifery education and practice were dominated by *doctors*. This, says Witz, was because 'at this historical juncture women's relation to the patriarchal capitalist state had *necessarily* to be mediated by men' (1992: 126).

Regulating the professions

Today midwifery is regulated by the UKCC (see Box 3.1). This body was established under the 1979 Nurses, Midwives and Health Visitors Act which, following the Briggs Report of 1972, sought to bring control of the professions in all parts of the UK under one body. Its aim was 'to make new provision with respect to the education, training and regulation and discipline of nurses, midwives and health visitors and the maintenance of a single professional register' (Department of Health 1979).

Four national boards were established and the Central Midwives Board (CMB), which had previously regulated midwifery, was dissolved. Such a move was contentious and was perceived by many to signal a loss of midwives' control over their own profession (Cardale 1990; Cronk 1990; Frame and North 1990). However, it had also been argued that the CMB had itself been ineffective in empowering midwives, since it was dominated by doctors (Cardale 1990; Robinson 1990; Royal College of Midwives, date unknown). The proposals for the new structure met with opposition and protest because nurses were seen to dominate. The Association of Radical Midwives (ARM) launched a campaign to resist the changes (Thomas 1979). It was suggested that there had been a lack of consultation with midwives and 'that those people in the highest echelons of midwifery and nursing held biased opinions concerning the proposed structure and its effects (at field level) because they were thinking and speaking from the standpoint of the bureaucrat' (Thomas 1979: 8).

A Midwifery Committee was set up within the council and each of the national boards, but interpretation of its role and the powers invested in it have been a continuing area of debate. Its very existence has been seen as something of a compromise (Ackerman and Winkler 1979; Cardale 1990; Cronk 1990).

Despite efforts to work within the new structure there was increasing dissatisfaction as changes were implemented of which midwife members of the midwifery committees did not approve. This was highlighted by a change in management structure at the English National Board for Nursing, Midwifery and Health Visiting (ENB) in 1988. Previously, midwifery education officers were accountable to a midwifery professional officer. From 1988 they were managed by the principal professional officer, who might not be a midwife. These education officers had responsibility for the validation and approval of training courses. Subsequently, education officers became 'generic' which meant that the non-midwife education officers would be able to make approval visits to centres of midwifery education. Approval had to be ratified by the Midwifery Committee who could make visits to a centre if they wished (ENB 1990). Midwife education officers could act only as specialist 'advisors' (Cronk 1990; Midwives Legislation Group 1990a, 1991). Also in 1988, the Midwives Legislation Group was set up by ARM to draw up alternative legislation and a new midwives act. Echoing the words of the Royal College of Midwives' president who was quoted as saying 'if we lose control of our education, we lose control of our profession' ARM took the view that this had indeed already happened. They campaigned for a new act (Midwives Legislation Group 1990b) which would provide for a separate midwifery body responsible for registration, education, training and monitoring standards of practice: 'in effect midwives will be answerable to their peers and no longer part of the UKCC' (Midwives Legislation Group 1990a: 12).

The argument for a new midwives act rests on the belief that midwifery is a profession, distinct from nursing (and medicine) and therefore should be self-regulating and have control over its own education. Where previously doctors dominated the CMB, nurses are seen to dominate the UKCC and midwives are a minority group, largely because of their numerical size. However, the Royal College of Midwives, the professional body, took the view that a new midwives act was 'neither practicable at the present time nor as yet proved desirable' (Royal College of Midwives 1991: 25). According to them, the statutory powers of the Midwifery Committee could secure an acceptable degree of control for midwives over their own practice and education *within* the structure established by the 1979 Act. In other respects the statutory arrangements were considered unsatisfactory and government-appointed management consultants noted evidence of 'tribalism' between the professions (Peat Marwick McLintock 1989). Doubt about the future role of the national boards was raised and professional control over nurse (and by implication, midwife) education was seen as under threat (Ratcliffe 1991). Under the 1992 Nurses, Midwives and Health Visitors Act the boards became government appointed bodies and the UKCC a directly elected body with responsibility for standards of education, professional conduct and practice. Against this background more recent developments in midwifery education may be understood.

The development of pre-registration midwifery education

During the 1980s a vigorous debate about the future of midwifery education emerged. This was largely a response to proposals made by the UKCC to reform both nurse and midwifery education. This period focused attention on professional conflicts that continued to shape the form and provision of education and training for both groups. Since registration began the length of midwifery education and training had become extended and there had always been a distinction made between direct entrants to the profession and nurse entrants (see Box 3.2).

Box 3.2 Policy developments in midwifery education 1903–91

1903   Registration begins
       3-month training for all entrants to midwifery

1916   6-month training for direct entrants
       4-month training for nurse entrants (3 months for those who had completed a gynaecology or children's nursing course)

1926   12-month training for direct entrants
       6-month training for nurse entrants
       (In 1929 fewer than 10 per cent of entrants were direct entrants)

1938   2 years' training for direct entrants
       1 year's training for nurse entrants
       Training divided into: Part 1 – 18 months for direct entrants
                                        6 months for nurses

Part 2 – 6 months for all candidates
(In 1940 1/1366 candidates for final exam was a direct entrant)

1949   Stocks report recommended cessation of direct entry route but this was not implemented

1968   Single period midwifery training introduced. Parts 1 and 2 phased out

1972   Briggs Report recommended all future midwives should be nurses and new curriculum design proposed for nurse and midwife education with 18-month common core foundation programme followed by 18-month specialist programme. Midwives would be expected to complete nurse training before going on to take a 1-year post-registration midwifery course. Led to Act of 1979

1981   3-year training for direct entrants
18-month training for nurse entrants
Changes implemented in line with European Directives 1980
(By 1983 only one 3-year training programme available in England)

1985   Royal College of Nursing Judge Report on nurse education developed Briggs' proposals. English National Board consultative document favoured development of direct entry midwifery courses. ENB's consultative document favours direct entry midwifery training

1986   UKCC Project 2000 proposals recommend 3-year curriculum with midwifery as a 'branch' of nursing. Links with higher education proposed and new courses to be at diploma level 18-month post-registration midwifery courses expected to continue

1987   Royal College of Midwives *The Role and Education of the Future Midwife in the United Kingdom* report advocates a 3-year curriculum for midwifery

1988   Radford and Thompson, funded by Department of Health and Social Security (DHSS) and ENB to examine how development of direct entry courses could be encouraged

1989   *Working Paper 10: Education and Training.* Department of Health provides pump-priming monies for seven new pre-registration courses with seven more planned in 1990

1991   *An Evaluation of the Implementation of Pre-Registration Midwifery Education in England* funded by the Department of Health (Kent *et al.* 1994)
(By 1993 when the evaluation was completed, 35 pre-registration programmes had begun)

Source: Radford and Thompson (1988); Kent (1995).

By 1983 there had been a decline in the number of 'direct entrants' to midwifery and only one midwifery school offered such a course. A number of explanations have been given for this. These generally focus on the lack of career opportunities for those without a dual qualification (both nurse and midwife registration) and on discrimination against direct entry midwives (Association of Radical Midwives 1980, 1981; Ball 1982; Downe 1986a, 1986b). According to some commentators, direct entry courses were of poor quality and the intense demand placed on service for practice placements in a three-year course were seen as contributing to this decline (Radford and Thompson 1988). Defenders of direct entry courses hotly contested the view that midwives trained in this way were in any sense inferior.

Against a background of patchy support for, and provision of, direct entry courses, discussions about the future of midwifery education during the 1980s became focused on the question of whether midwives should train first as nurses. This was related to dissatisfaction with the position of midwives in maternity services discussed in Chapter 2. It was suggested that:

> dissatisfaction with the current role and status of the midwife underlies the resurgence of interest in direct entry: the direct entrant, so long seen as an inferior breed of midwife (compared to her jointly qualified sister), is now proposed as the guardian of the future of midwifery. [Direct entry midwives] are thought to be less tolerant of the encroachment of the medical model of sickness into normal maternity care, less willing to conform to the norms of the doctor-nurse relationship, and therefore more able to accept the responsibilities demanded of an independent practitioner.
>
> (Curtis 1986: 4)

According to Curtis, writing in 1986, this 'U-turn' indicated the midwifery profession's efforts to reassert a separate *identity*. It seemed that direct entry was to be supported on ideological grounds since it asserted a distinct identity for midwives and produced a practitioner who was better suited for 'independent' practice. While the 1979 Act was seen by critics as marking a particular stage in disenfranchising midwives, later events in the education arena represented a more fundamental attack. Specifically, the UKCC Project 2000 proposals (UKCC 1986a, 1986b) were controversial since they appeared to subsume midwifery into the nursing profession. Many midwives saw this as an attack not only on their ability to control their profession, but also on their professional identity.

From 1985 there was a shift in thinking about nurse and midwifery education that was to develop into an energetic debate about the relative merits of the direct entry route. The publication of the Royal College of Nursing's *Commission on Nursing Education* (the 'Judge Report') (1985) and the 1985 ENB consultative document *Proposals for Change* in education and training marked a significant turning point in England. The key proposals were:

- There was to be a shift in all nurse education to focus on 'health', and 'direct entry' to all specialities in nursing: mental nursing, mental handicap, paediatric nursing, general nursing (hospital), general nursing (community), *midwifery* and health visiting.

- All courses would be of three years' duration.
- There would be a common core in health.
- Collaborative links would be established between schools of nursing and midwifery and institutions of higher education.
- Students would be supernumerary (extra to the paid workforce).

The ARM was supportive of these proposals in principle (MacKeith 1985) and there was widespread agreement that a common core programme could be acceptable and that direct entry midwifery should be increased (Radford and Thompson 1988).

Project 2000 and the midwife

Initially the ENB proposals were welcomed as recognition of the claims already made for direct entry midwifery courses. It was even suggested that the proposals for nursing followed the midwifery example. However, in the Judge Report the relationship between midwives and nurses was considered more 'prescriptive' as it appeared to subsume midwifery as a specialism of nursing (Newson 1986a, 1986b). The UKCC Project 2000 documents followed and it provoked a vigorous response from midwives (UKCC 1986a, 1986b). A two-year foundation course was proposed followed by a one-year 'branch programme' (this was later reduced to 18 months). Five branches were identified, one of which was midwifery. The reduction of midwifery content to one year was considered a retrograde step by some commentators (Scruggs 1986) and the ARM stated that they wanted no part of it (Hughes and Parker 1986). Others pointed out that the proposals stressed the need to see each qualifying programme as of three years' duration (MIDIRS 1986). Midwives were asked to consider an experiment of three-year midwifery programmes and a new list of competences set out in new training rules, which would supersede the existing midwives' rules. The UKCC accepted 'that midwifery is a profession different from, but complementary to nursing' and claimed that Project 2000, with the common foundation programme, 'offers many of the attractions that the direct entry lobby seeks and avoids some of the disadvantages' (UKCC 1986a, para. 6: 33).

Some of the UKCC Project 2000 reforms were accepted – notably the links with higher education, the focus on health, the supernumerary status of students and shared learning (joint lectures) between professions *where appropriate* (Newson 1986a, 1986b; Royal College of Midwives 1986; Tickner 1986). However, many of the proposals were considered unacceptable. The Royal College of Midwives recalled the legislative framework of the midwife's role to justify rejection of the notion of a 'new animal' in midwifery as envisaged by the UKCC. In addition the existing competences of the midwife were thought by them to be undermined in the new proposals. In so far as Project 2000 was seen to represent a fundamental attack on midwifery as a separate profession, it was rejected outright. The distinctiveness of the midwifery profession was expounded vehemently by a midwife who later took up post as the chief midwife at the Department of Health (and who commissioned the evaluation of pre-registration midwifery education in 1991) (Kent *et al.* 1994):

Firstly midwifery is a separate profession *not* the seventh branch of nursing. Second, there is already a three-year training course for midwives based on agreed EEC directives and geared to the midwives' needs, producing a practitioner on qualification. Beyond doubt there is a need to increase the number of direct entry courses available to train midwives. What is proposed may be right for the future preparation of nurses but not for midwives . . . *Wake up!* We must not allow ourselves to be engulfed and swamped by these proposals, which would not produce the midwife practitioners we need and would, once and for all, see the demise of midwifery as a separate profession.
(Greenwood 1985, cited in Curtis 1986: 22, emphasis added)

Opinion was divided because others saw the changes as providing midwives with new opportunities (Newson 1986a, 1986b; Roch 1986; Pope 1987) which, if carefully negotiated, could further enhance midwifery education. Notably, ARM proposed that midwives should go it alone and the need for an alternative plan to Project 2000 was considered necessary (Association of Radical Midwives 1986; Dickson 1986; MacKeith 1985).

The Royal College of Midwives did produce its own report in 1987 entitled *The Role and Education of the Future Midwife in the United Kingdom*. This did not address explicitly the issue of direct entry but outlined a midwifery curriculum and endorsed the principle that midwifery programmes should be three years in duration. *The Role of Education* neither ruled out the possibility of a midwifery course as part of Project 2000, nor advocated a quite separate training for midwives. The report was ambivalent in this respect, though it did reinforce the statutory responsibilities of the midwife, and the distinct professional identity of the midwife. The need to retain 'the separate and distinct competencies for midwives' was emphasized (p. 6). No reference was made to the shorter post-registration course for nurses (Radford and Thompson 1988) though the Royal College of Midwives had expressed support for its continuation elsewhere (Tickner 1986).

Importantly, the distinctiveness of the midwife as 'guardian of the normal' was weakened by the 'health focus' of the new nurse practitioner envisaged in Project 2000. Clearly, to pursue the argument that midwives were distinct because they emphasized 'health' and 'normality' could not, on its own, support the case for a separate midwifery course. So the debate shifted emphasis to the independence of the midwife practitioner and her specific level of competence, responsibility and decision-making as the key features of a midwife's professional identity. Strategically this was successful as Project 2000 dropped midwifery from the branch programme. On the surface at least it seemed that midwives' voices, although divided on some issues, had been heard. Yet from the evidence of earlier arguments for direct entry and the legal definitions of a midwife (UKCC 1991a), midwives' ability to identify themselves as professionals relied on definitions of 'normal' and 'abnormal', 'health' and 'illness' (see also Curtis 1986). This suggests that the professional identity of the midwife was indeed under threat. In the autumn of 1986 in England the ENB sought midwives' opinions on developing separate direct entry midwifery courses, and widespread coverage in the midwifery press reported enthusiasm for more of these (*Midwife, Health Visitor and Community Nurse* 1986; *Mid-wives' Chronicle & Nursing Notes* 1986; Scruggs 1986).

Promoting direct entry

The ENB and the DHSS subsequently funded a study to promote *Direct Entry: A Preparation for Midwifery Practice* (Radford and Thompson 1988). This study followed earlier research conducted by the ARM direct entry working party (Association of Radical Midwives 1986; Downe 1986a, 1986b, 1987). Evidently there was a commitment by the ENB and the then DHSS to promote direct entry courses. In 1987 the DHSS had recommended to regional health authorities that they should have at least one such course. The one-year study was to assess the factors affecting the implementation process (Radford and Thompson 1988). Promoting the courses proved too difficult for the researchers who stated that intervention by the statutory bodies or 'a consensus amongst midwives as to the future direction of the profession' was needed (Radford and Thompson 1988: 8). It seems that initially such a consensus had been assumed by the ENB at least, if not the researchers, and although there was widespread support, the profession was still divided. Radford and Thompson reported that support for direct entry was primarily on *ideological* grounds among midwife educators, while regional health authorities were seen as concerned with pragmatic issues centred around workforce issues and training costs. They concluded that 'the whole issue is linked to a bid to re-establish the midwife as a practitioner with a distinct professional identity' (Radford and Thompson 1988: 104). At the same time some midwife teachers were reported as favouring the Project 2000 proposals in a modified form rather than separate training for midwives. In many respects Radford and Thompson's report was unsatisfactory in that it did not address fundamental issues about direct entry as a preparation for midwifery but rather, under the direction of the ENB and DHSS, took these for granted.

Soon after, the 1989 *Working for Patients: Education and Training Working Paper 10* stated 'the Government wishes to see an expansion of direct entry midwifery, which is more cost-effective in the long run' (Department of Health 1989b, para. 6.7). Funding for training was redirected to regional health authorities who would become purchasers of midwifery education. Workforce considerations (the need to ensure a supply of suitably qualified midwives) and the potential cost advantages of pre-registration midwifery courses were given as the principal reasons for these developments (Department of Health 1989b, para. 6.4). The links with higher education were to be strengthened for all health courses. The case for change was couched in 'pragmatic' terms and invoked none of the ideological reasons for pre-registration midwifery education. Professional ideologies were subsumed under managerial imperatives.

Pump-priming monies were released by the Department of Health to set up new pre-registration midwifery programmes at 14 sites, originally intended to be located in each of the regional health authorities. From this time what had previously been called 'direct entry' courses were formally redefined as 'pre-registration programmes' which would be at diploma or degree level and have links with higher education. Students would be supernumerary and each programme would be at least three years in length. However, the earlier debates about direct entry courses and the controversy around the Project 2000 proposals informed attitudes to these new programmes. In addition, research monies were made available to evaluate the new courses and a national three-year project carried out (Kent *et al.* 1994). Research into the new programmes has continued, supported by the ENB and the Department of Health (Eraut *et al.* 1995; Gerrish *et al.* 1996a, 1996b; Phillips *et al.* 1996; Fraser *et al.* 1997).

So far I have outlined the changes in midwifery education from the time when handywomen gained experience through practice and had no formal training, to the development of the professional midwife. Early midwifery courses continued to emphasize practical skills and schools of midwifery were located in the hospitals, close to the practice setting. Training was mainly on the job, and was later combined with time spent in the classroom. Theoretical knowledge became increasingly valued as midwives were expected to be educated professional women, though their position remained subordinate to the doctors. In practice it is often obstetric-led hospital policies which determine what midwives can do (see Chapter 2). This can lead to midwives, as practitioners legally accountable for their own practice, having to defend decisions that were not their own (Oakley and Houd 1990). Midwifery education may be characterized as initially based on an apprenticeship model and later a vocational one. Benoit (1989), in her study of midwives in Newfoundland and Labrador argued that the latter of these is most effective in producing 'competent and committed professionals' (p. 160). She was also critical of university-based education. Her view was that university educated midwives need closer supervision in practice and that the occupational role became more narrowly defined. According to Benoit the university education midwife became more of a technician with less autonomy or professional control. Although cautious about generalizing her findings to other midwife groups, Benoit took the view that university education weakens professional control and reduces practical experience. The relevance of Benoit's findings for the UK may be limited but she did raise some interesting questions about the effects of reorganizing midwifery education in another context. University-based midwifery education has now become widely available in the UK and the impact on midwifery practice is still being assessed.

Degrees of freedom – the integration of health professionals in higher education

Between 1989 and June 1993 35 new pre-registration midwifery programmes were set up in England. By October 1998 there were 44 programmes in England, one in Wales, six in Scotland and none in Northern Ireland (see Table 3.1). This indicates a growing support for the pre-registration approach that was encouraged by the changes in policy already outlined.

However, in England the implementation of the new programmes at the local level revealed a number of interesting processes and issues which

Table 3.1 Number of pre-registration midwifery programmes in the UK for 1998

	England	Scotland	Wales	Northern Ireland
Diploma (higher education)	22	6	1	0
Degree (3-year)	13	0	0	0
Degree (4-year)	9	0	0	0
Total	44	6	1	0

Sources: Figures obtained from ENB Careers Service (September 1998); SNB (October 1998); WNB (October 1998); NIB (October 1998).

were reported on at that time (Kent *et al.* 1994). Evidently a variety of institutional forms developed which related, at least in part, to local organizational politics. However, these local changes were largely informed by the broader ideological debate about the relative merits of the earlier direct entry courses. For many midwives the legacy of the past was strong and some were sceptical that the new programmes of education could produce high-quality midwives. They believed that all midwives should train as nurses first and many were themselves dually qualified. Others saw the opportunity to develop a pre-registration midwifery course as a chance to strengthen their position locally, to improve the profession's standing and secure a future for midwives which would enable them to practise as 'independent, autonomous practitioners'. They emphasized the distinctiveness of the midwifery profession and hoped to recruit a new type of student who would be committed to a distinctive midwifery approach. The pre-registration midwife could, like the earlier direct entrants, be expected to stand up to medical practitioners, assert the professional values of midwives and treat pregnant women as normal and healthy. In contrast to post-registration student midwives there would be no need to encourage them to see pregnancy as a healthy, natural process, for the new student would not have been socialized into thinking about illness or pathological problems.

Cooperative links with a university, polytechnic or college of higher education were essential to meet the requirements for the new courses which could be at diploma or degree level (ENB 1990, 1993a). The shape and form of links made with higher education varied according to local conditions and where the midwives felt most willing to go. For some this meant physically relocating midwifery staff to the higher education institution, while others remained in the former hospital-based school of midwifery and students or lecturing staff moved between sites for teaching and learning. Concurrent changes in higher education, which from 1992 created the new universities, contributed to a time of transition and instability. Research by Kent *et al.* (1994) which looked at pre-registration midwifery programmes in England, and by Phillips *et al.* (1996) in their study of nursing and midwifery degree programmes, points to the diversity of institutional forms and the importance of local circumstances in shaping them.

Curriculum changes

Midwifery teaching contracts were reissued and in some cases there were redundancies, while others remained anomalously on NHS contracts. Lecturers from higher education were, for the first time, called upon to teach student midwives (and nurses). Non-clinical specialists, most often in the social, behavioural and biological sciences, were expected to contribute to the development of a curriculum that was still determined by the criteria of the profession's regulatory bodies, the ENB and the UKCC (Eraut *et al.* 1995). At the same time the universities' own criteria for validating and approving courses had to be met. Midwives' success in negotiating what, for them, was an acceptable outcome was diverse. In some cases they maintained considerable control over the curriculum content and the management of the programme. In others, restructuring of management hierarchies did not always enable midwives to maintain the upper hand (Ho 1991). Increasingly, fears were expressed that midwives were in danger of losing control of their education to an extent that had not been previously envisaged (Downe 1990). As the curriculum broadened to include new subject areas and greater numbers of non-professionals taught on the new courses, professional ideologies were threatened and undermined.

In particular, relationships between midwife educators and their clinical colleagues working in midwifery services were affected by these changes. Where previously they had often enjoyed close working relationships and shared the same physical work environment, increasingly teaching activities became relocated in classrooms and institutions away from the hospital. Although some groups were able to maintain strong links and service colleagues had input on the planning and validation of the new courses, others became more educationally led and contact between education and service managers decreased (Kent *et al.* 1994). This suggests some similarity with Benoit's (1989) findings in Newfoundland. Changes were compounded by the development of the market in education as newly-formed NHS Trusts became purchasers of courses provided by institutions of higher education. In the early days this split between financial and managerial control of midwifery education caused confusion and increasingly midwives had less control over education planning (Kent *et al.* 1994). Many midwives regarded the increased distance between education and service and the weakening of links as a retrograde step, and as undermining professional solidarity. It also affected the ability of clinical midwives to gain insight into the educational programme and into their role as mentors to students on placements, planned as part of the new courses.

Concern was expressed about the need for the approved midwife teacher, responsible for the midwifery education programme, to secure her position in the restructuring (House of Commons Select Committee 1992; Warwick 1992; Silverton 1996). Yet, in the face of new lines of managerial control and accountability this was deeply problematic. The ENB supported their position arguing for representation 'within the institution's policy making machinery' (ENB 1992) and produced guidelines, rather belatedly in 1993, when many amalgamations had already taken place (ENB 1993b). The Royal College of Midwives (1993) also reiterated the importance of recognition of the special requirements for midwifery education. The power and role of the ENB in validating and approving courses was also under threat in the face of new, and unfamiliar, university regulations and procedures. As a result, midwife teachers found themselves caught between two validating bodies and contrasting cultures.

Relationships between midwives and nurses

Within the newly amalgamated institutions relationships with nurses were also contentious. In some cases midwifery and nursing schools had already joined together prior to establishing links with higher education. In others, midwives had maintained a distinctive midwifery school (though many small midwifery schools had already joined together). This influenced negotiations about new links and in turn about the shape and content of the new curricula. 'Separate midwifery schools and colleges began from a different power base' though increasingly the ability of midwives to remain separate from nurses became more difficult (Kent *et al.* 1994, vol. 1: 33). At issue here were professional boundaries between nurses and midwives and different ideas about the new curricula. Given the controversy that had surrounded Project 2000 there continued to be divisions and conflicts around the content and design of the new courses. Midwifery students on some of the new courses were, after all, to receive joint lectures with nursing students on Project 2000 courses. Others had shared learning with medical and dental students, nursing degree students and occasionally with other student groups. There were different views of the need for practical placements in nursing areas and debate about the overlap between 'nursing skills' and 'midwifery skills'. Increasingly, there was widespread agreement that midwives did not need to train as nurses, but uncertainties about the merits of the pre-registration courses among some midwives continued. Solidarity with nurses at the institutional level was in some cases a matter of 'practical expediency' (Kent *et al.* 1994) in situations where the small number of midwives made political representation in higher education particularly difficult. Critics however argued against such alliances and regretted the closer connections with nursing courses (Downe 1990).

A professional project

A principal benefit expected as a result of the development of pre-registration midwifery courses was an increased credibility and status for midwives as a professional group. Consistent with earlier credentialism, a higher education award of a diploma or degree was thought by many to signal greater authority for the profession. Support for pre-registration midwifery education, seen as a professional project, assumed that benefits could accrue to midwives under the new structures. Perhaps surprisingly at this time, the Royal College of Midwives' director of professional affairs, Rosemary Jenkins, suggested in 1993 that midwives, in seeking professional status for its own sake were in danger of becoming 'elitist' and 'protectionist'

(Jenkins 1993). She proposed that the profession should be cautious about the effects of increased 'intellectualism' associated with the move into higher education, and instead combine the benefits of the apprenticeship model of practice-based learning in an 'intellectual apprenticeship model'. Following other writers on the professions (for example, Abbott and Wallace 1990; Hugman 1991), she challenged the uncritical acceptance of professional ideologies. More recent evidence suggests that expectations have been modified.

By entering the arena of higher education midwives have been faced with other traditions and the effects of changes taking place in the university sector. Problems in the early days of pre-registration midwifery education with unfamiliar regulations and procedures of the university set the scene. In addition new conflicts and tensions have emerged. Within the university sector existing hierarchies between science-based disciplines, social sciences, academic and vocational courses have structured the experiences of midwife teachers and students (and their nursing colleagues). The contractual relationships and working conditions of midwives compared to other academic staff have also caused tensions. Where health service salaries have been honoured the new lecturers have been seen as an expensive burden; in other cases new contracts with lower salaries have been offered. Contrasting levels of pay and the length of study leave and holidays highlight differences between staff groups and mark out new boundaries between them. Phillips *et al.* (1996) report on the changing context of academic and professional values. They argue for a managerial strategy to unite professional and academic cultures and point to the way in which each is 'positioned' by the other. They contrast rigid and hierarchical relationships in nursing and midwifery with 'relationships of trust' in the academy. Drawing attention to the impact of changes in higher education they highlight the challenge to the midwifery (and nursing) professions to develop research.

A research-based approach to practice

Increasing tension between the demands of teaching and research characterize higher education in the 1990s. Changes in the funding of higher education through the Higher Education Funding Council (HEFC) have led to assessment of the research output and activities of universities. In the first assessment exercise of 1992 'nursing', which included midwifery, achieved the lowest rating compared to 70 other subjects (Phillips *et al.* 1996). In 1996 many more nursing departments were entered in the research assessment exercise (RAE) and although the majority of them were rated 1 or 2 (1 being the lowest and 5 the highest), 11 out of 36 departments scored a 3a or 3b (Kitson 1997). This indicates a significant achievement. Given the relatively short history of nursing and midwifery research and the short time the professions have had to develop a research culture in higher education, the difficulties facing nurses and midwives to develop research are considerable. Pressures on midwife lecturers to develop research skills, gain research qualifications and establish research profiles are intense. Alison Kitson, a leading nurse researcher argued in 1997 that a national strategy for developing research was needed, together with investment, support and training for nurse and midwife researchers. She says there has been a lack of coordination and planning to assist with the transition of nurse (and midwifery) education into higher education. She called for monies to develop an infrastructure and the potential for research. Despite real difficulties in managing time for teaching, research and clinical practice, there has been a proliferation of midwifery publications (for example, Bryar 1995; Hunt and Symonds 1995) and some departments have developed research programmes and encouraged midwife researchers.

In Chapter 2 I contrasted the medical and midwifery models of care, and drew attention to the absence of formal, codified knowledge for midwifery practice. Now that midwives are in the university sector there are both opportunities for such codification but also inherent difficulties. A focus of debate has been on the relationship between theory and practice. These have frequently been thought of as in a dichotomous (and hierarchical) relationship to each other. Theoretical knowledge, although often held in higher esteem in academic circles, has in the past been treated with caution by midwives who seek to emphasize their *practical* competences and the 'art' of midwifery. Efforts to promote research in midwifery and the development of midwifery theory (Henderson 1990; Bryar 1995; Kelly 1997) may be seen as synonymous with an increased *scientization* of midwifery. Certainly such a move has been generally welcomed by nurses (Salvage and Kershaw 1990; Chapman 1992; Kent *et al.* 1992) and midwives but this signals a fundamental shift for midwives who traditionally have emphasized their relationship to women and their experiential and practical knowledge. The extent then to which theorizing experiences or codifying practice is either desirable or realistic is contentious. Tacit knowledge is defined precisely as that which cannot be codified – it is tacit (Collins 1985). Therefore while midwives, like nurses and other professional groups, have extolled the virtues of developing 'reflective practitioners' (Schön 1983, 1987) the limitations of this are not always recognized. Moreover, the distinctive professional identity of midwives, it has been argued, is contingent on a special relationship with women. How far that relationship could be changed by a growing allegiance to scientific discourses and a new style of research-based practice is an open question.

A new type of midwife?

Louise Silverton, Director of Education and Practice Development at the Royal College of Midwives, following Jackson (1993), questioned the view that education is necessarily 'a good thing' and that more education for midwives is better. She argues that 'midwifery is such a practical profession and one where status should not depend solely on academic achievement' (Silverton 1996: 83). She believes that a rise in the academic level of midwives for the sake of strengthening opposition to the medical profession is inappropriate and that the test of its value is how far it improves maternity care. For this reason, like Jackson (1993) and Jenkins (1993 see above) Silverton asks whether midwives with a higher education will produce 'a midwifery elite rather than preparing the midwife to be "with woman"?' (Silverton 1996: 84). Her view is that the experienced midwife should be able to achieve graduate status, but the pre-registration midwife needs to prioritize practical experience in the clinical area. Kirkham (1996) is also cautious about the consequences of professionalization and its impact on midwives' relationships with women. She seems to recognize that certain knowledge cannot easily be codified and that emphasis on rule-following and procedures may be detrimental to the quality of care. Rather than acting from insecurities about their professional status, Kirkham wants to see midwives developing knowledge which enables them to develop powerful alliances with women and to share knowledge with them.

In contrast Henderson, another midwife educator, says 'the move into higher education is both stimulating and challenging and I believe that it will greatly enhance midwifery education by encouraging a spirit of enquiry that will inevitably lead to a more *empowered* workforce' (Henderson 1994: 224, my emphasis). Her vision is a midwife with a broader knowledge base and 'highly developed skills who will be able to practise independently or within the NHS' (p. 224). For Henderson, an expert and knowledgeable midwife produced via the new diploma and degree programmes will be more able to work as an equal partner with the doctor. Accordingly the new midwifery curriculum may be seen as enhancing midwifery practice but also potentially changing midwives' relationships with others. These contrasting views of the pre-registration approach point once again to the close connection between knowledge and power and the importance attached to a professional identity. For students on these courses, these tensions are apparent in the way they talk about their experiences of becoming midwives.

Becoming a midwife – a politics of identity

Studies of occupational **socialization** in the professions have a long history which Dingwall and Lewis (1983) trace back to the 1930s. Since the 1960s there have been well-known studies of student doctors, nurses and health visitors which have drawn attention to the ways in which these professions reproduce themselves through programmes of education and training (Becker *et al.* 1961; Dingwall 1977; Simpson 1979; Melia 1981, 1987). Few studies of midwifery have been done. In a study of post-registration student midwives in the UK, Davies and Atkinson (1991) report the emphasis on the ways students learn the job and 'cope' with the day-to-day work of midwifery but also how the students' 'individual self-image and sense of identity' was threatened. They say that over time new 'identities begin to crystallise, perspectives are laid down and [coping] strategies begin to emerge' (Davies and Atkinson 1991: 120). As in Melia's study of student nurses (1981, 1987) the emphasis is on the ways in which students learnt the job and 'coped' with the day-to-day work of midwifery but reference is made to a more fundamental change in *identity* and self-image. This process is seen to occur over time, to produce a once and for all transformation of the students and the development of an altered self-image and a new identity – the professional identity of a qualified midwife.

My own research explored how students on the new pre-registration midwifery programmes developed a professional identity (Kent 1995, 1999). Rather than seeing the educational programme as simply the acquisition of knowledge and skills I highlight the significance of professional *discourse* and ideologies. I see the construction and articulation of identity as a continual process of *becoming* a midwife, as a *discursive process* whereby students learn to mobilize competing, and sometimes contradictory, accounts of what it means to be a midwife. The students themselves, however, have a view of a midwife identity as fixed and unitary.

Identity politics

Students frequently articulated differences between midwives and nurses and midwives and doctors while similarities between midwives and nurses were often ignored. They could be seen to engage in a form of **identity politics**, defining and policing the boundaries between those who are midwives and those who are not. At the same time they highlighted similarities between themselves and the women they cared for, claiming solidarity with them. 'Working with women' defined for them what it means to be a midwife (Kent 1995). In the context of the pre-registration midwifery programmes the differences between professional groups remained central. These students, often with no previous background as health professionals, adopted many of the ideas and much of the thinking of the midwifery profession and positioned themselves in the higher education setting in certain ways.

Identity politics rests on a personalizing of politics and *identification* or sense of belonging to a group. Hall (1992) explains how, as a new social movement, feminists appealed to women to challenge their social position and the formation of sexual and gendered identities. In a search for unity and solidarity feminists emphasized this identification as part of an oppositional strategy to overturn patriarchy and capitalism. In this conception of the feminist subject, identity became a fixed and unifying concept. Similarly, the students' conception of a midwife subject was fixed and unitary. Identity politics, then, may be seen as located historically within the modern world where ascription of male and female roles has been characteristic of industrial society (Giddens 1991; Beck 1992; Hall 1992). The position of midwives as a professional group relies on the ascription of a specified role and naturalized identity.

Emphasizing practical knowledge

At the centre of the development of a professional identity for midwives is an emphasis on the differences between midwives and doctors. Yet paradoxically the identity of the midwife is contingent on that of the medical practitioner for she became defined as that which he was not, as 'other' and 'different'. The demarcation of their professional roles outlined above defines what it means to be a midwife. Students recognized this and reiterated the view that midwives were 'autonomous' practitioners in their own right. The legal framework was used as a justificatory strategy to assert the midwife's status and her role, demarcating her sphere of responsibility. As Witz (1992) and Oakley (1989) argue, this was a gendered identity, and the rationality and scientific knowledge of the doctor was set in opposition to the practical and experiential knowledge of the midwife (see Chapter 2). In relation to nurses other differences were emphasized.

Guardians of the 'normal'

The identity of midwives is considered distinct from nurses in two important ways. First, midwives have a statutory responsibility for pregnant and labouring women (see p. 50) whereas the nurse is seen as acting under the direct supervision of the doctor. Second, the midwife is concerned with 'normality' and 'health' (see Chapter 2) whereas the nurse is seen as traditionally oriented towards 'abnormality' and 'illness'. Flint, a well-known midwife, criticized the notion that midwives should train first as nurses saying there was no more justification for this than the idea they should train as florists (Flint 1986). The student midwives instrumental in setting up the ARM were keen to support direct entry midwifery courses as a means of distinguishing between nurses and midwives and ensuring that midwives were enabled to develop and use their skills to the full. An ARM working party (convened in 1983) set themselves the explicit task of promoting the direct entry route to midwifery qualification. They argued that the direct entry midwife had a distinct approach to midwifery (Association of Radical Midwives 1980, 1981; Downe 1987). The identity of the midwife seemed inseparable from the means by which she was educated since caring for the healthy, rather than treating the pathological, 'comes naturally to the direct entrant' (Ball 1982: 12).

Much has been said about the extent to which students prepared via the pre-registration route will be different from previous midwives and a long-term evaluation of this has now begun (Fraser et al. 1997). At the time of my research however these students argued that distinctions between them and nurses were important and they were therefore critical of the nurses they came into contact with during their course. For them, shared learning with nurses and placements in nursing areas simply did not acknowledge these differences enough. Since these learning experiences have been included in the educational curricula the strategy of highlighting differences between nurses and midwives has been only partially successful in influencing changes in midwifery education, as already described.

Learning to practise

Despite the move to higher education the students valued most highly the practical placements (especially with community midwives). They saw themselves as 'clinically based' not as university students and preferred to 'keep our identity as a practical profession' (Kent 1999). At the same time though, their ability to 'fit into' the clinical environment was a problem for them and at other times they were critical of midwifery colleagues. It was then that they identified more closely with the women in their care, positioning themselves between the professional midwife and the woman (Kent 1999). They expressed solidarity with the women, drawing attention to the ways in which the maternity services failed to meet women's needs. They attached great importance to the *emotional work* of midwifery and an ethic of care that highlighted their connection to other women. This feature of midwifery work will be discussed in the next chapter, but here it is seen as an important way in which midwives construct their identity. At other times, the students described the effects of an alienating hospital environment as disempowering midwives and so they aligned professional interests with the interests of the women who used their services. An emancipatory discourse underpinned their criticisms of the hospital midwifery service and arguments for greater professional status for midwives were considered of mutual benefit.

Identity and difference

Identity politics depends on the identification (and fixing) of subject positions. In feminist theory this has increasingly been criticized as exclusionary and unacceptable in so far as it denies differences *within* categories and is based on an epistemology and politics of naturalized subjects (see Chapter 6). Instead, subjectivity may be seen as fluid and mobile (Ferguson 1993) and politics as 'a struggle for the very articulation of identity, in which the possibilities remain open for political values which can validate both diversity and solidarity' (Weeks 1994: 12). Accordingly I see the students as moving between subject positions, as women, as students, as midwives. In so doing they specify these positions and situate themselves in relation to other positions which they themselves constitute – men, women, qualified staff, nurses and doctors. These moves, as well as being constituted in relation to 'others', are tied to specific institutional contexts and local situations. So in the context of the hospital ward, differences between students and qualified staff had salience, while on other occasions relationships to doctors were seen in opposition to midwives. During the placements in nursing areas identifications as midwives, distinct from nurses, were mobilized. In the university their identity as *professional* midwives was prioritized in relation to other university students and again where nurses were present. In other 'care' contexts their identification as women took priority, as they aligned themselves with the 'cared for' rather than the uncaring professional midwife.

Conclusions

This chapter has developed a sociological perspective on midwifery education in the UK with a focus on England. In order to understand the complex issues underlying the education and training of today's midwife

I have analysed issues at three levels. At the policy level I have shown how the transition from handywoman to professional midwife is characterized by efforts by midwives to secure occupational territory and status for themselves. This has been closely related to disputes with the medical profession and its demarcationary strategies. By the 1980s midwives had been partially successful in securing a degree of autonomy and self-regulation though within strictly defined limits. Education and training, as part of a 'credentialist tactic' (Witz 1992) continued to be important throughout this period. Since the 1980s however, professional conflicts with the nursing profession have also been significant both in shaping the regulatory bodies and education programmes. Major reforms to nurse and midwifery education have characterized the 1990s and led to new conflicts and tensions. Specifically, the ability of the midwifery profession to control its own education has been undermined.

At the institutional level, links with higher education have weakened the position of midwife teachers and changes in funding have meant that they have little financial or managerial control. Alliances with nurses have been contentious and this has been reflected in the design and content of educational curricula. The value of nursing placements for pre-registration midwives is still being debated and although the competences of the midwife, in law, remain the same, the inclusion of a wider range of subjects has occurred. Opinion is divided about the value of this broader knowledge base and worries that these new midwives will be too intellectual and lack practical experience have raised questions about the assumptions underpinning the new courses. While diplomas and degrees have been expected by some to give midwives greater freedom, power and control (in accordance with credentialist thinking), others are uncertain about the benefits. Could, for example, the highly educated midwife become elitist and distant from the women she cares for? Or will the new programmes produce a better educated midwife and more competent practitioner? Are professional values important after all?

In an educational context where academic values are emphasized, professional aspirations appear under threat from both directions. As professionals, or as academics, midwives are under pressure to develop research and theorize their practice. The growing emphasis on evidence-based practice is intended to promote the application of research findings in the practice setting and to link together theory and practice. However, we may be witnessing a *scientization* of midwifery as attempts are made to codify and systematize formal midwifery knowledge. Of itself this appears to contradict claims to be a practical profession 'with women' (though only in so far as theory and practice are considered separate). In their evaluation of the outcomes of pre-registration midwifery programmes Fraser *et al.* (1997) conclude that the new programmes are providing an effective preparation for midwifery practice. They also say that these newly-qualified midwives demonstrate a good understanding of midwifery research. However they believe that a new model of competence is needed since 'there was no commonly shared definition of a competent midwife at the point of registration' (ENB 1997: 4).

In my research, professional values were seen as being at the centre of a midwife identity and students on the new pre-registration courses continued to see these as important. They identifed strongly, much of the time, with the professional values of midwives, emphasizing their distinctiveness from nurses and from doctors. They also did not see themselves as university students. In addition, they aligned themselves 'with women' believing that what is in the interests of midwives will also benefit women. They aspired to become independent, autonomous practitioners and invoked the legal position of midwives as justification for this. The view taken here is that students are not simply socialized into an occupational role and do not assume the identity of the midwife as a cloak. Rather, they develop over the course of their educational programme an ability to mobilize competing and sometimes contradictory accounts of what it means to become a midwife. Becoming a midwife is seen here as a discursive process. Students' identity as midwives is constituted in a political struggle for midwives to be recognized as a powerful social group. This struggle continues and in the next chapter I examine further the reasons why midwives, as a predominately female occupational group, have been positioned in a sexual division of labour that continues to disadvantage them.

Summary

- Professional education is important to midwives not least because it controls who may practice and helps to set standards for practice. In this chapter I have discussed how this process of controlling access to professional education and practice is a political struggle.

- In the 1990s the professional agenda has often been framed in terms of the need to develop and extend the knowledge base of the midwife. Some argue that the movement of midwifery education into higher education in the last decade provides an opportunity to produce a new type of midwife.

- Today's midwife will be expected to develop a research–based approach to practice, and to be able to theorize practice. Changes in the midwifery curriculum have led to the inclusion of social sciences and biological sciences, and new forms of midwifery knowledge are being developed. My argument here, though, is that since knowledge and power are intimately connected the implications of these changes are complex.

- Using a sociological perspective to analyse the changes leads to a view that midwives have also been engaged for many years in a struggle to obtain professional recognition and status. This struggle has been influenced by relationships with other professional groups, notably doctors and nurses. In order to set boundaries around the work that midwives do they have attempted to define a distinct and separate professional identity.

- This process of identification has shaped policy debates around the regulation and control of education programmes, and conflicts at the local level.

- Students on the earliest pre-registration midwifery programmes were seen to be actively involved in constructing their identities as midwives. They sought to emphasize differences between themselves, nurses and doctors. I argued that they were engaged in a form of identity politics.

- It is not my intention here to imply that the move of midwifery education into higher education has been motivated simply by self-interest. Neither do I wish to deny that it may be beneficial to women who need a midwife. Instead my aim has been to show how the development of new forms of midwifery knowledge cannot be separated from an analysis of power relations. Knowledge is not a neutral commodity, as is sometimes assumed. From a sociological perspective knowledge always constructs and is tied into power relations. Attempts therefore to theorize midwifery do inevitably imply a transformation of what it means to be a midwife and to be 'with woman'.

Discussion points

- In what sense did the early midwives acts represent a working out of the struggle of midwives for autonomy and power?

- How have professional conflicts continued to shape midwifery education and practice?

- To what extent do the links with higher education provide the promise of professional freedom for midwives?

- Why has the legal status of the midwife continued to be important for shaping the education debate?

- Are midwives trained by the pre-registration route different from those who are already nurses?

- What is meant by identity politics?

Further reading

Abbott, P. and Meerabeau, E. (1998) *The Sociology of the Caring Professions*, revised edn. London: University College London.
Hall, S., Held, D. and McGrew, T. (eds) (1992) *Modernity and Its Futures*. Cambridge: Polity Press.
Hugman, P. (1991) *Power in the Caring Professions*. London: Macmillan.
Witz, A. (1992) *Professions and Patriarchy*. London: Routledge.

FOUR

MIDWIFERY AS 'WOMEN'S WORK'

Introduction

In the last two chapters I have outlined developments in maternity services and the midwifery profession. My discussion has explored the relationship between knowledge and power, the professionalizing strategies of midwives and recent changes in midwifery education. Here I consider the links between knowledge, power and skill. I shall examine the idea that midwifery is 'women's work'; that what midwives do has been commonly seen as an extension of what women do 'naturally'. Becoming pregnant and giving birth is often regarded as the natural function of women's bodies. Emphasis on the reproductive activity of women and assumptions that 'motherhood' is a natural and normal state for women has had both material and ideological effects.

Historically there has been a division between *reproduction* and *production* in modern industrial society. Women have been understood as primarily associated with the first of these, involved in the processes of giving birth, caring for children and reproducing labour power in the private sphere of the home and family. In contrast, men have become associated with the public sphere, with production and paid work. A **sexual division of labour** has characterized western society where these divisions are mapped onto men and women, though more recent evidence suggests that some changes are occurring. Sociological analysis of women and work points to the ways in which, in modern industrial society, women's ability to participate in the labour market has been structured by gendered processes.

Well paid and high status jobs for women have not been easy to access because of underlying beliefs about what constitutes appropriate activities for women. In the nineteenth century, certain occupations such as midwifery, nursing, social work and teaching came to be regarded as acceptable jobs for single, middle-class women. These women could afford to live independently. Historically, in the UK, social and employment policies have regarded women as dependent on husbands for financial support, and higher wages for men (the family wage) were accounted for in this way. Single women were expected to get married or continue to be supported by their parents (fathers). Even today the position of women at work relates to their position in the household (private sphere), and a sexual division of labour where women (especially married ones and women with children) are commonly constrained by domestic commitments which limit their ability to undertake paid work. Discussion of women and work therefore needs to examine the connections between these two spheres.

The next chapter will focus more specifically on motherhood while the focus of this chapter is on women as midwives, undertaking 'women's work'. There are four key questions I aim to address here:

- What does it mean to 'care' for pregnant women?
- Is caring 'natural' or learnt?
- Why is caring work generally low status and low paid?
- How do the answers to these questions help to explain the organization of maternity services, the work midwives do and the care pregnant women receive?

The concept of care is important for both midwifery practice and mothering because in certain respects midwives are seen to 'care' for women in similar ways as mothers 'care' for children. We shall see how the *identity* of midwives and mothers is closely tied to the idea that they are 'carers'. But what does it mean when midwives say they care for labouring women? How may we understand their role as carers and supporters of women and the importance of 'emotional work'? Since this is what midwives argue is distinctive about their work we need to understand how caring work is gendered.

The gendering of work is a complex process. I shall draw on an extensive literature from the sociology of work, feminist theory and research on care in order to understand why midwifery work, as women's work, is consistently undervalued. Carers in employment are often low paid, and in the home caring work is usually unpaid and carried out by mothers, daughters or wives (Oliver 1983; Pascall 1986; Dalley 1988; Lewis and Meredith 1988; Ungerson 1990). Care work is generally regarded as unskilled and of low status. But how are concepts of skill socially constructed and how is work gendered? Midwifery, because of its association with reproduction, has been of relatively low status compared to medicine. Midwives have struggled to define themselves as skilled workers and expert helpers.

In an influential book edited by Finch and Groves (1983), Hilary Graham (1983) outlined how care has two dimensions to it. On the one hand it refers to relations between the carer and cared for, the *feelings* the carer has (seldom is this seen as a reciprocal relationship but more of that later). On the other hand it has a material or *economic* basis and refers to the provision of goods and services. Graham's discussion then examines the idea that caring is a *labour of love*. I shall consider both aspects here and more recent work that is critical of this division. A major strand of this discussion is the organization of work and the **labour process**. The material or economic aspects of 'care' and midwifery 'work' are of central importance. In addition however, it is the moral basis of social relationships, the *ethic of care* that underpins much caring work. Feelings of attachment to others, respect for others and a sense of personal and social responsibility are distinctive features of certain caring relationships. Midwives, by seeing their work as 'emotional labour', draw attention to this and emphasize their connection to other women.

The implication of this analysis is that first, only when the values of care and reciprocity are seen as central to those of social justice, responsibility and community can a better future for both midwives and mothers be attained. This in turn would assist with a revaluing of caring work and a recognition of the importance of social support for health. Such a revaluing also requires changes in the *material* circumstances of women. Only with higher rates of pay for the labour women perform, as both mothers and workers, can the damage and oppressive effects of the current unequal situation be addressed.

This chapter is organized in three sections. Section one summarizes the theoretical debates relating to gender and work. These include references to economic and social theories of the labour market and labour process in capitalist society. Feminist revision to earlier theories examines the concept of **patriarchy** and the extent to which **capitalism** intersects with **gender relations**.

Section two turns to a discussion of the NHS as a particular sector in the labour market economy. The employment of women in the NHS is of interest in that it contributes to a further understanding of **occupational segregation**. More specifically the historical division of labour between medicine and midwifery is examined. This enables me to extend the earlier discussion in Chapters 2 and 3 and consider why midwifery is still regarded as 'women's work'.

The final section looks at aspects of midwifery work and the relationship between midwives and women by considering what 'caring' means.

The public and private spheres

In a review of theoretical approaches to studying work in modern society, Crompton and Sanderson (1990) explain how earlier class theories failed to take account of gender. Class analysis and **stratification theory** provided a conceptual framework for thinking about production in capitalist society. In Marxist theory, *class* was seen as an historical social division which gives rise to conflict and change. Relations of production are central to this division and workers are seen as exploited and oppressed through the accumulation of profit (capital) from their labour power. An employment contract ties workers to their employers who in turn benefit from their labour. Workers are regarded as 'free' to enter into the employment contract. These Marxist views have been contrasted with Weberian conceptions of class that identify status and occupation as linked to class position (Porter 1998). Feminists have argued that women were excluded from these analyses.

Women in the labour market

There is extensive evidence that even today women tend to occupy lower paid, lower status jobs. Various theoretical explanations have been put forward to account for the position of women in the labour market and Bradley (1989) gives a good summary of these.

According to traditional economic theory, women possess less **human capital** (knowledge and skills) due to interruption of their careers to have children. Human capital theory has been criticized because it cannot explain the position of women without children or those who do not take career breaks. It also fails to take account of the skills and knowledge women acquire through 'caring' for children, other 'dependants' and domestic labour. Evidence shows that even where women have accrued considerable education, skills and experience they are relatively disadvantaged.

New home economics outlined by Sue Hatt (1997) assumes that because a man's wage is usually higher than a woman's there are greater costs to him staying at home than if the woman remains there. Hatt explains that in economic terms the 'opportunity costs' of women entering paid work have increasingly acted as a constraint on their participation. Since women are usually lower paid than men, households are financially better off when men earn the wages and women stay at home. Hatt draws attention to structural inequalities in the labour market and in the household which have restricted and limited women's participation. Goods and services produced in the household, by women, are not costed into the national income accounts or assigned an economic value. In effect, what women do at home by way of labouring to cook meals, cleaning and caring for children, older, disabled or sick relatives, is invisible and undervalued. By contrast the productive activities of men in the labour market are seen as valuable and contributing to the economic wealth of our society.

Because some women's participation in paid work is commonly interrupted by childbearing and childcare, women do not have the same chance to develop the skills and experience recognized by employers to develop their careers, or gain promotion through continuous service. Therefore traditional explanations of the ways in which jobs come to be filled by men, such as human capital theory, are inadequate for explaining why women are disadvantaged. What is important here is that those skills which women do acquire are not regarded as human capital by employers or most economists. A feminist economic analysis tries to revalue women's labour but does not explain what kind of powerful interests are served by maintaining the status quo. As Hatt (1997) points out, the problem with this analysis is that it relies on a circular argument about the value of women's labour in the economy, and rather than explaining *why* men's wages are higher than women's, takes this wage gap as a starting point.

Another suggestion is that women tend to 'crowd' into certain sectors of employment where employers are more willing to employ them or where jobs are compatible with women's domestic responsibilities. This results in an over-supply of labour and lower wages. In contrast the resources and skills possessed by men are regarded as scarce and therefore command higher wages. Once again this, says Bradley (1989), is unsatisfactory because it gives no explanation of why *employers* act in this way. Neither does it examine the constraints on women's participation in the labour market.

In the past women have been seen as a 'reserve army of labour' able to move in and out of the labour market since they are occupied with domestic commitments (Bruegel 1979). This influenced the demand for their labour and reinforced their role as mothers, reproducing and caring for the labour force in the private sphere of the home, and encouraged economic dependency on wage earning men. So feminist economists have argued for a reframing of economic theory to take account of the domestic work women do, seeing the unpaid activities of women in the home as of economic importance (Gardiner 1997; Hatt 1997). Sociologists have maintained that housework and mothering are indeed *work* (Oakley 1974a, 1974b). Explanations about why men and women tend to occupy different jobs and about changes in the patterns of employment are also needed.

Occupational segregation in the labour market

Studies have examined the ways in which certain jobs are regarded as 'men's work' and others as 'women's work' (Crompton and Mann 1986). A sexual division of labour in employment is seen as structuring the opportunities available to women. According to dual labour market theory (Barron and Norris 1976) women and men participate in the labour market in quite distinctive ways. In effect the labour market is seen as segmented, with women (especially those with children) moving in and out of quite different jobs from those of men. **Horizontal occupational segregation** describes the patterns of employment showing that women are more usually employed in lower paid, low status jobs. But even in jobs where women outnumber men (e.g. nursing), men occupy more senior jobs and there is **vertical segregation** (Hugman 1991). A feminist analysis draws attention to the ways in which women are systematically excluded from certain jobs and disadvantaged at work, and how both economic and *cultural* factors interrelate.

Patriarchy and capitalism

Feminist opinion about the causes of inequalities in the labour market is divided. Gender theory tells us *who* fills the jobs that are created under capitalism. Sylvia Walby (1986) adopts a feminist, Marxist perspective. In her discussion of patriarchy she says women are systematically excluded from certain jobs and access to decent pay and working conditions. This in turn is seen as forcing them into marriage and dependency, doing unpaid work in the home. She argues that the nineteenth century was characterized by private patriarchy and the twentieth century by public patriarchy. Women became doubly disadvantaged by the drive for cheap labour and their continuing subordination to men. For Walby, patriarchy and capitalism intersect and coexist as two separate systems that interact. Patriarchal institutions such as trade unions have acted, using different patriarchal strategies, to subordinate women in jobs that are graded lower than similar ones done by men, or to exclude them from paid employment in the first place. Walby argues that the interests of capital and of men compete for the benefits of women's labour, explaining the patterns of women's employment and the reasons for the marriage bar on certain jobs. Until the post-war years, once married, middle-class women were expected to leave their jobs in nursing and midwifery, and in other areas of employment married women were sacked. Women's labour power is simultaneously appropriated by men in the home in a patriarchal mode of production and in the workplace by patriarchal strategies of exclusion and segregation. Rather than seeing women as disadvantaged in the labour market *because* of their domestic role, Walby's analysis focuses on patriarchy as a system that operates both in the workplace and at home.

In contrast, Rosemary Crompton (1990) argues that capitalism describes the way in which industrial societies are structured and labour relations produced, but that the absence of gender in class theory does not negate class as a general idea. She says that 'patriarchy' was developed as an alternative explanation to class theory but she does not see patriarchy as a universal concept or process. For Crompton, patriarchy is one aspect of gender relations rather than a *system* and she does not believe that Walby provides an adequate theory of patriarchy. Crompton argues instead for an approach to occupational segregation that is multi-factoral. She examines how a variety of theories are useful in different case studies. She says that both economic and social factors are relevant and have effects in different institutional contexts. Sex-typing of jobs, 'crowding' of women into low paid jobs, patriarchal exclusionary practices and other features of the labour market are all seen by Crompton as contributing, in a dynamic way, to the division of labour.

Sexuality, gender, family and the labour market

Lisa Adkins (1995) argues that earlier feminist accounts of this **dual systems approach** which see patriarchy and capitalism as relatively distinct processes are inadequate. In her critique of Walby (1986), and Hartmann (1979, 1981) she argues that capitalism is gendered, and following Pateman (1988) she maintains that 'a worker is a gendered phenomenon' (Adkins 1995: 43). According to her analysis, women are not 'free' to enter into the wage contract under capitalism because they are subordinated to men. Capitalism therefore is patriarchally constituted since the constitution of labour power for men and women is different. Her argument is that men and women:

> are different sorts of workers. They do different sorts of work even when working alongside each other, and have different relationships of and to production. Moreover the gendering of production means that men occupy a structurally more powerful position in all these various areas of employment, a position from which they can control and appropriate some of the products of the work of women.
>
> (Adkins 1995: 148)

By drawing attention to the connections between sexuality, the family and the labour market, Adkins demonstrates how 'economic' and social relations are constitutive of each other. Gender, rather than being external to the labour market, *is produced by it.* Gender relations are produced as part of the work (see Box 4.1).

Sexuality therefore structures the labour market and a compulsory heterosexuality is reinforced. Following Rich (1983) who argues that compulsory heterosexuality organizes and structures women's labour inside and outside the labour market, Adkins says 'economic and social factors are all arguably sexual in that they may be connected to heterosexuality' (1995: 35). Sexuality and the family have both economic and social significance in contemporary patriarchal capitalism.

Service work as sexual work

What is particularly interesting about Adkins' (1995) analysis for this discussion is the way in which she draws attention to the specific features of *service work as sexual work.* Similarly, in a discussion of nurse stereotypes Jan Savage (1987) highlights the sexual work which nurses perform and how relations with patients are structured by widely held beliefs about women who provide services. As Adkins argues, integral to this kind of work is the implicit, if not explicit, assumption that women (and nurses) are available to provide sexual services. However, unlike Adkins, Savage does not see this as part of the labour process but proposes that

Box 4.1   Women workers in the tourist industry providing 'sexual services' and the implications for other women's jobs

In Adkins' (1995) example, women in the tourist industry performed 'sexual services' as part of the job. Being attractive, looking the part and being willing to accept treatment as a sexual object by customers and co-workers were *requirements* of the job. Failure to perform in this way meant a woman was not doing her job properly and might face dismissal.

In her analysis, sexual work has economic value, for example, it brings customers into a pub where, it is generally believed by company managers, men prefer to be served by a woman. Wives of pub landlords and hotel managers were therefore performing sexual services as part of their *husbands'* jobs. The wives themselves had no employment contract but a marriage contract bound them indirectly to their husbands' employer. This, says Adkins, shows that earlier feminist analysis which see the family as a separate (private) sphere from the (public) labour market is inadequate. Reporting on the staff training programme of tourist workers, she recalls how 'people skills' and 'caring for guests' were seen as of primary importance. Given the way in which all manner of service jobs routinely sexualize women's work, and the ways in which women are routinely sexualized and constituted as different sorts of workers compared with men through this sexualization, it seems that the specific conditions attached to women's employment at these two worksites, far from being atypical, may be one of the constitutive features of 'women's work'. Indeed, even studies of women's manufacturing or professional employment suggest similar processes in operation.

stereotypes in the media and elsewhere must be challenged because 'they may prevent us [nurses] from realising opportunities to acquire a powerful voice in the promotion of health' (Savage 1987: 95). She recognizes that these nurse stereotypes weaken nurses' position and power, but does not offer an analysis of how and why they are produced. If, however, we see the powerful interests of men and capital structuring the nursing process, the causes of these problems begin to come into view. Relations of production in the health service therefore are of particular interest for this discussion of midwifery as women's work and can be related back to conflicts already highlighted between midwives, doctors and nurses in Chapters 2 and 3.

Different kinds of workers

To summarize the discussion so far, there is widespread evidence to show that men and women do different kinds of jobs and are different kinds of workers. Explanations for this include a variety of approaches that

emphasize economic and/or social processes. Dispute about the extent to
which there is an overarching theory of the labour process includes a
discussion about the relative merits of a class-based analysis and/or patriarchy as systems of oppression and exploitation of women by men. Dual
systems theorists see both as operating while others, such as Adkins (1995),
seek to integrate the economic and social spheres, arguing they are constitutive of each other. Gender is seen by some to be external to the labour
market but interacting with it, but Adkins says gender is produced *by* the
labour market. Gendering the labour process is important for understanding why certain occupations such as midwifery come to be regarded as
'women's work'. Moreover, the idea that women's jobs are less skilled may
be seen to be a product of both ideological and material processes rather
than an intrinsic quality of the work they do. It is because *women* do this
work that it is relatively low paid and of low status. Historical and contemporary accounts of relations of production within the health service
and the medical division of labour are better understood in the light of
gender theory.

Occupational segregation in the NHS and the medical division of labour

Within the NHS women workers have made important contributions.
However, occupational segregation has structured the opportunities
available to them, their pay and working conditions (Miles 1991; Doyal
1994; Davies 1995). Women today are frequently employed as cleaners,
administrative staff, nursing auxilliaries, nurses and midwives. In contrast
men enjoy more senior positions as doctors, consultants, health service
managers and technicians. Such divisions are constructed around the use
of technologies and different forms of knowledge. We saw in Chapter 1
how the division between the work of obstetricians and midwives is constructed around the prioritizing of scientific rationality and technological
management of childbirth in contrast to the practical and experiential
knowledge of midwives. Obstetricians have come to be regarded as highly
skilled and of high status in contrast to the lower status and less skilled
midwives.

Table 4.1 shows the segregated workforce in the NHS. The majority of
nurses, midwives and health visitors are women. In contrast the majority
of doctors and dentists are men. Women make up the largest number of
direct care workers in the NHS, outnumbering men by four to one. A
census of the nursing, midwifery and health visiting professions in 1991
(see Table 4.2) showed that the pattern of women's participation in nursing work also differs from that of men. A large number of qualified nurses,
midwives and health visitors are considered 'economically inactive'. This
group comprises mainly married women. Leder (1995) says single women
are more likely to be working compared to married women. Women with
young children are most likely to be out of paid work. Forty-one per cent
of women who had left the profession said this was to raise a family while
no men gave this as a reason for leaving. The main reason men left the
profession was to take up other employment.

Table 4.1 NHS hospital and community health services directly employed staff by main staff group and by sex (whole time equivalents), September 1992

	Nursing, midwifery and health visiting	Medical and dental	Professions allied to medicine*	Total direct care staff
Female	335,150	14,290	65,830	415,270
Male	43,640	32,930	23,990	100,560

* including other scientific, technical and professional staff.
Source: Department of Health (1992).

Table 4.2 Numbers of men and women under the age of 55 working in nursing, midwifery or health visiting in 1991

	Working in the profession	Working outside the profession	Economically inactive	Total
Men	2,607	989	273	3,869
Women	28,524	6,365	6,730	41,619
Total	31,131	7,354	7,003	45,488

Source: Leder (1995).

Professions and patriarchy

Anne Witz's (1992) discussion of the sexual division of labour in medicine and professions and patriarchy provides a useful analysis of how the development of midwifery as a profession has been shaped by both patriarchy and class interests. Following Hartmann (1979), Cockburn (1983, 1985) and Walby (1986, 1990) Witz argues for an approach to women and work which incorporates both concepts of patriarchy and capitalism. Importantly for these writers, women's position in the labour market cannot simply be read off their position and status in the family, as we have already seen. Rather, patriarchy may be seen as an historical and materialist system which operates in different institutional contexts. So, drawing on Walby's work, patriarchy and capitalism are seen as interacting, but autonomous, systems. According to Witz's reading, Walby is arguing that the direction of influence is from the labour market to the family rather than the other way round (Witz 1992). Patriarchal relations are constituted in the workplace through strategies of exclusion and segregation. Historically, women are subordinated by the actions of male craft unions and employer practices that systematically exclude them from certain jobs and attribute to them sex role stereotypes. Women then, according to this analysis, face a double jeopardy as class and gender intersect. As outlined in Chapter 2, Witz explains how the power of the medical profession to set limits on midwifery practice was related to its position as a male dominated institution and its relationship to the state. Witz attributes the success of the medical profession's demarcationary and exclusionary strategies to both powerful class interests and gender relations. These are produced through what she refers to as the twin processes of *professionalization* and *masculinization*.

Witz (1992) says a fundamental shift and restructuring of the market for medical services, together with new forms of occupational control, resulted in the marginalization and exclusion of women practitioners. Where previously there was a preference for the services of a local 'wise woman' emphasizing familial and neighbourhood relations, the growth of industrial capitalism created a different market for medical services. This in turn had the effect of shifting these services from the hands of women healers to medical men. At the same time an increasingly specialized division of labour 'also contributed to the demise of female medical practice, because [it] severed gender specific routes of access to and involvement in the activities of family business' (Witz 1992: 81). It is this movement of medical services from 'the private domestic to public market' which disadvantaged women practitioners (Witz 1992: 82). Men were better able to represent their interests in the public sphere and develop institutional forms of occupational control while, Witz says, women were less able to organize themselves. She gives a fascinating account of how such changes were nevertheless contested by women in the nineteenth century and later how the relations between doctors and midwives were constructed.

The social construction of 'skill'

In Chapter 2 I discussed how the ability of doctors to gain control over the provision of maternity services forms the background to conflicts today. Importantly their success also rested on arguments that technical and theoretical knowledge are superior to the practical knowledge of midwives. Accordingly, the way in which 'skills' and knowledge are defined is central to inequalities in the labour market. Yet, as Witz (1992) and other social theorists argue, the ability of certain groups to sustain these kinds of arguments rests on other economic and social factors. Access to institutional forms such as the university, professional associations and the state facilitated the entrenchment of male power in the medical arena. By controlling entry to a profession (both medicine and midwifery), the intention is to increase the market value of certain skills and knowledge.

As I discussed in Chapter 3, the recent movement of midwifery into higher education as part of a credentialist strategy is expected by some parties to increase the status, value (and pay) of midwives. This may be seen as a response to earlier 'deskilling' of the midwife when registration began in 1902. In essence the market for midwifery services was segmented into those provided by midwives at lower cost and those provided by the doctor. Witz's (1992) thesis is that both groups engaged in 'professional projects' that were gendered. Doctors exercised 'demarcationary strategies of exclusion' which produced a division of labour between obstetrics and midwifery and set strict limits on midwifery practice. Midwives emphasized education and training, securing a form of occupational control through closure that did not threaten the dominant role of the obstetrician but enabled midwives to assert a professional identity for themselves.

The kinds of strategies available to occupational groups are, according to this analysis, contingent on **gender relations**, so midwives accommodated the medical profession and conceded power to them in order to secure a degree of autonomy for themselves. Strategies on both sides mobilized *gendered discourses* about 'men's work' and 'women's work'. Midwifery was 'women's work' and therefore regarded as less technical and less skilled. Abnormal or complicated pregnancies requiring skilled and technical expertise remained within the control of the obstetrician and were seen as 'men's work'. The division of labour and occupational boundaries are therefore supported and maintained through 'gendered discursive as well as gendered closure strategies' (Witz 1992: 127).

Skill – reskilling or deskilling?

In a more recent discussion of the nursing profession Thornley (1996: 165) explores the idea that the state has been able to play on divisions within nursing and 'the nebulous character of skill in nursing' to employ cheaper labour in the NHS. She sees divisions between auxillary nursing staff, enrolled nurses and registered nurses as class based and segmented by race and gender. Many of the auxillary and nursing staff in her study were part-time and not eligible to belong to the professional organization of the Royal College of Nursing, so they were recruited to the trade unions. This Thornley sees as a form of 'grade dilution'.

Thornley outlines the bargaining which has occurred during the 1980s and 1990s to include these staff in pay review body assessments. Subsequently she argues that although Project 2000 and the movement of nurses into higher education was intended as a form of professional closure, it has in fact resulted in new forms of grade dilution. Managerial strategies have included reducing the number of qualified nursing staff and employing 'support workers' at much lower cost to perform services which were previously regarded as nursing work and done by qualified and student nurses. This point is also made by Walby *et al.* (1994). In effect Thornley (1996) says this amounts to a 'deskilling' of nursing work made possible because 'skill' is constantly being redefined.

According to Thornley's analysis the professionalizing strategies of nurses have emphasized the technical aspects of their work and underplayed 'caring' work and experience since these have less value and command lower status and pay. Thornley shows how 'skill' becomes redefined through the interactions of managerial strategies to reduce labour costs and increase control, relating in turn to the effects of action by professional bodies and trade unions.

Skills and the midwife

The discussion above about the connections between 'skill' and 'caring work' raises some interesting questions for midwives who, like nurses, have moved into higher education and anticipate a revaluing of their skills following *Changing Childbirth* (Department of Health 1993), as indicated in Chapters 2 and 3. In practice, training and employing midwives is cheaper than training and employing obstetricians and they may benefit from a deskilling of obstetricians. However, it also seems likely that, like nurses, they will need to underplay the caring aspects of their work and the emotional labour they perform, and emphasize instead their technical competence. This, paradoxically, goes against the arguments for a midwifery-led service. Hunt and Symonds (1995) draw attention to this paradox, pointing out that it is commonly argued that midwifery practice in the hospital setting has deskilled midwives. This is contentious, for as Hunt and Symonds suggest, midwives have learnt new skills in the hospital and acquired technical competence in practices that had previously been the domain of the doctor.

By moving the site of production (birth) out of the hospital, it has been argued that midwives will be able to rediscover traditional midwifery skills and be reskilled, but not necessarily revalued. Hunt and Symonds (1995) rightly draw attention to the flawed logic here. Historically, traditional midwifery skills were not valued and when skill is seen as socially constructed depending on who does the job, there is little to suggest that any reskilling will take place. Midwives are usually women and women's work almost by definition is unskilled. Hunt and Symonds' discussion brings into dispute the potential effects of *Changing Childbirth* (Department of Health 1993) (see Chapter 2). It cannot simply be assumed that midwives will enjoy new power and status, become reskilled and better paid. Instead, midwives' ability to secure greater control over birth is likely to be associated with a deskilling of obstetricians and a cost-cutting exercise in maternity services.

As Hunt and Symonds (1995) suggest, new-found 'autonomy' may 'become redefined within the existing set of ideological assumptions regarding both the primacy of the public over the private sphere and also the gender-based hierarchy of "skill"' (p. 153). They also express concern that changes in the delivery of midwifery services and specifically certain forms of 'team midwifery' which include on-call and 'flexible' working hours will have the added effect of excluding women with domestic commitments (see also Sandall 1996, 1997). Certainly the evidence of other studies, such as that by Thornley (1996), indicates that downgrading of tasks is likely to be associated with the shift from hospital-based, obstetric-led care to home-based, midwifery-led care. It is less likely that restructuring the organization of maternity services will result in new recognition for midwifery and a revaluing of 'women's work'.

In their later book, *The Midwife and Society*, Symonds and Hunt (1996) outline the growth of managerialism in the NHS since the 1970s and suggest that this represents a fundamental threat to professional power and greater control by the state (see also Elston 1991; Gabe *et al.* 1994; Davies 1995). Certainly the downgrading of midwifery (and nursing) work runs counter to any claims for enhanced professional status. However, Symonds and Hunt's analysis fails to consider the extent to which the professions mediate state power themselves, regulating and controlling social behaviour through professional-client relations. Although increasingly professions have been called to account and subjected to tighter financial control their continued efforts to maintain and secure autonomy may be seen as both commensurate with the 'new wave management' to which Walby *et al.* (1994) refer, and to tensions within it.

Governance and the restructuring of the NHS

Walby *et al.* (1994) analyse the nursing and medical professions in a changing health service and explore how tasks are divided between them through complex negotiations, conflict and cooperation. They suggest that the way health work has been organized is changing. By seeing these divisions as both related to professionalizing strategies and changes in the organization of work they explore how nurses and doctors work together. They consider how increased efficiency drives in the 1980s that emphasized throughput of patients have impacted on health work. In addition more recent 'new wave management' ideas characterized by local decision making by semi-autonomous teams and by tighter managerial and financial control have created additional tensions in the workplace. The introduction of greater accountability through mechanisms such as clinical audit and the implementation of evidence-based practice are part of the changes being implemented (Ackers and Abbott 1996). The effects on nursing were considered ill thought-out and nursing work was undervalued (Davies 1995).

Walby *et al.* (1994) suggest that old forms of work organization (along Taylorist production lines) led to fragmentation and increased specialization of tasks. Ward teams were loosely organized around different 'time-space geographies' of nursing and medicine. The study by Walby *et al.* (1994) of acute surgical wards showed that there has been increased pressure on ward teams arising from the restructuring of management, and efficiency drives. This has resulted in fragmentation and poor communication which is associated with 'a disintegration of the ward as an organic unit' (Walby *et al.* 1994: 121). However, rather than seeing interprofessional relations as fixed and rigid, as in earlier analyses, Walby *et al.* conclude that the professions of medicine and nursing are both complementary and competitive. In their study doctors supported nurses becoming more skilled especially in areas which doctors would continue to control. Boundary disputes were most likely to occur between junior doctors and nurses but in general doctors were pleased to offload skilled work, previously done by junior doctors, to 'their' nurses who were members of the ward team they controlled.

According to the analysis by Walby *et al.* (1994), the divide between 'care' and 'cure' is not a straightforward one and in any case is in a state of flux and change. Moreover, they suggest that there is no simple hierarchy between the professions as some theorists have proposed (see also Annandale 1998). In different situations doctors and nurses become allies against, for example, the general managers, senior nursing staff or consultants (see also Cox 1991; Elston 1991). The challenge facing the NHS now is, according to Walby *et al.*, to find ways of managing professionals who have different traditions of self-governance. They see doctors as having:

> a mode of governance which has similarities with that advocated by new wave management. Nursing does not have the autonomy that is associated with the traditional form of a profession, and has had a form of governance more consistent with Taylorism, though recent changes demonstrate a movement away from this.
>
> (Walby *et al.* 1994: 155)

So in their view, though nurses are highly skilled they lack autonomy and are rule bound, task orientated and hierarchically organized. They say this is changing with the introduction of primary nursing, team nursing and Project 2000.

The introduction of general management has had different effects for the two professions. Doctors have been able to reposition themselves within the new structures. In contrast nurses have, according to some commentators (Strong and Robinson 1990; Davies 1995), been displaced and have lost power. New wave management theory emphasizes local decision making by relatively skilled workers in teams, and cuts across the interprofessional (hierarchical) relationships between nurses and doctors. In certain areas, doctors continue to seek control over the nursing services but such conflicts and tensions are influenced by other changes. Similarly, boundary disputes between doctors and midwives and the division of labour between them may be seen as constrained and reshaped by managerial strategies for reorganization. As already suggested a significant improvement in working conditions for midwives seems unlikely.

New practices implemented under *Changing Childbirth* (Department of Health 1993) must be understood within the wider context of managerial thinking in the NHS. In so far as greater autonomy for midwives at the local level is commensurate with devolved decision making then midwives might expect their efforts to succeed. However, such gains will no doubt be tightly constrained by financial and centralized control over other aspects of their work. The breaking down, or blurring, of boundaries between their role and that of obstetricians is likely to be offset by the ability of general managers to mediate and control interprofessional relations. Reorganization in the NHS has had complex effects on the organization of service work and the role of health care professionals (Davies 1995) but there is little research on midwifery work practices from a sociological perspective (Sandall 1995, 1996, 1997). The next section examines more closely both the nature of the 'caring relationship' (the relationship midwives have 'with women') and the organization of midwifery work.

Caring work as women's work – a labour of love

Students on pre-registration midwifery courses emphasized that what is distinctive about midwifery work is the emotional labour or emotional work which they do (Kent 1995, 1999). Providing support for women and being 'with women' was what they believed marked out midwifery care from what obstetricians do. Midwives frequently make this distinction as part of a professionalizing strategy, as we saw in Chapter 2. Ann Oakley (1989) reinforces this idea that midwives *care* for women and *love* them. Her research on the effects of social support was based on the principle that care has important benefits for pregnant women (Oakley 1992). These claims are premised on certain assumptions that merit closer attention. In what sense do midwives 'care' for women and what can we understand by the notion of 'emotional labour'?

One underlying assumption appears to be that women are most able and better equipped than men to care. On occasion midwives appear to mobilize **essentialist** ideas that women are *naturally* caring and good at care. It seems that notions of *femininity* and *masculinity* are embedded within these claims. This has implications for arguments about whether men should become midwives and the ways in which those that do may be regarded. A second assumption is that as women, midwives are equal to, and able to care for, all other women. They emphasize similarities between themselves and the women in their care (Kent 1999) and fail to examine important differences between women, and the ways in which social divisions within the caring relationship may be significant (Graham 1991). So for example the fact that midwives are commonly middle class, white, and (now) university educated women has implications for their relationship with black, working-class, lesbian and disabled women.

Concepts of care

Jennifer Mason discusses the concept of care and highlights different dimensions of caring, distinguishing between material and moral aspects. Referring to the work of Hilary Graham (1991), she says, 'the conflation of "caring for" with "caring about" in, for example psychological explanations of why women care, obscured the labour intensive nature of women's caring work – seeing it as simply part of women's caring psyche' (Mason 1994: 3).

Mason recognizes the importance of acknowledging that caring is indeed *work*, as does Lee-Treweek (1997) in her discussion of nursing auxillaries' work in a nursing home. In contrast to commonly held expectations these nursing auxillaries had instrumental views of their work. For them it was a job which in some cases they hated but which provided them with a small income. They were resistant to certain aspects of the work and selective in their response to the 'needs' of 'patients'. As with other studies of nursing (Melia 1987) getting the job done, maintaining the routines of the institution and managing the patients were their priorities.

Midwifery *work* is also about 'managing' women, routinized care in hospital, shift work and controlling access to information and resources (Kirkham 1983, 1989). The midwifery process may be understood as comprising a set of formal procedures for monitoring the health and labour of the pregnant woman. Pregnancy and childbirth are divided into stages, and care has been organized around these by setting up antenatal clinics, delivery suites and postnatal wards. Midwives, though generically trained, have specialized in community midwifery, antenatal care, delivery and neonatal care. Students' learning has been divided along similar lines (Kent *et al.* 1994). Work routines such as drug counting, ward reports and allocation of 'case' loads are all elements of the organization of midwifery work.

Sheila Hunt's ethnography of midwifery (Hunt and Symonds 1995) provides interesting insights into the workplace and the organization of hospital-based midwifery work. Presented as features of the organizational culture her account reveals how midwifery work is tedious, laborious, dirty and ritualized. Bloodstains on midwives' uniforms were considered symbolic of a hard day's work well done. Patients who were identified as 'dirty' were regarded with disdain. Midwives distanced themselves from these women until they were 'clean' (Hunt and Symonds 1995: 90). There is little here to support the idea that these *workers* 'care about' or have strong feelings of attachment to these women. Indeed intimacy with clients or hospital patients is frequently frowned upon and discouraged.

The student midwives in my study referred to the 'special relationship' they had with women but also said that being a midwife was more than being a friend (Kent 1995). *Caring for* someone does become construed as *caring about* them even when, as Lee-Treweek (1997) points out this does not necessarily follow (Ackers and Abbott 1996). Hunt's study provides evidence to the contrary. She draws attention to the ways in which midwives made a 'moral evaluation' of women on admission to the hospital. Patients were assessed 'according to their language and social competencies' and their social position (Hunt and Symonds 1995: 91). Clearly, relationships between midwives (carers) and the women they 'care' for are more complex than is sometimes assumed.

Emotional labour

According to Jeff Hearn (1987):

> the main role of the semi-professions such as midwifery and nursing [Hearn argues] is to take on the emotional labour involved in professional-client interaction . . . People-work such as midwifery, nursing, social work and counselling is thus seen as a 'natural' arena for the female qualities of caring empathy and patience and so structurally these jobs remain female-dominated and of a lower status and prestige.
>
> (Hearn cited in Hunt and Symonds 1995: 21)

It is the midwife who can be expected to comfort the bereaved woman after a stillbirth. Yet at the same time Hunt and Symonds (1995: 82) describe the relationship between the midwife and the labouring woman as like parent and child with the midwife adopting a position of authority and power using terms of endearment such as 'sweetie pie', 'lovey' and 'poppy'. Although some women in Hunt and Symonds' study accepted this as common practice among midwives, it can also be considered patronizing and offensive. The quality of the relationship between the woman and midwife, as with all caring relationships, is therefore problematic – it is an economic relationship and one of *power.*

The midwife as health professional mediates the woman's access to resources and provides her with goods and services. At the same time professional *discourses* construct the experience of pregnancy and childbirth through the use of specialized, technical language (for example, foetal cardiac arrythmias, post partum heamorrhage). Much has been said about the importance of women knowing their midwives (Flint and Poulengerie 1991). But Hunt and Symonds (1995) say that a successful labour is not seen in terms of the process itself, the quality of the birth experience, or even the quality of the relationship between the midwife and the woman. Rather, success is commonly defined as the production of a live, healthy baby. This brings into doubt the value midwives attach to emotional work. So while they say 'birth has much to do with emotional labour and is often about the intense professional-client interaction described by Hearn (1987)', Hunt and Symonds (1995: 84) do not really analyse the significance of this, given their findings. Indeed their study indicates that the criteria for assessing the quality of midwifery services are very similar to those used by obstetricians. *Biological* indicators are used rather than social ones and form the basis for measuring outcomes. In this regard these midwives reproduced and perpetuated a *biomedical* view of pregnancy and childbirth.

Social support

In contrast, Ann Oakley's study (1992) aimed to examine the impact of *social* relationships on the health and well-being of pregnant women and their babies (see Chapter 2). She framed her work against a background of earlier studies on social support, pointing out that social support is not a new concept and has for some time been seen as health-promoting. Her review of the growth of social support studies highlights methodological problems and the difficulties of defining what it means, or how it works.

There has been a distinction made between studies that suggest that the quantity, or size of social networks relates to physical health, and those that suggest that the quality of relationships is linked to psychological health. However, this dualistic thinking originates in a binary divide between certain kinds of measurable effects and others, and between different methodological traditions. Oakley argues that 'the history of medicine is the history of the importance to health of social support' (1992: 32), and that well-known 'placebo effects' can be explained by the idea that the doctor-patient relationship has therapeutic value as opposed to the use of 'treatments' such as drug therapy which do not. Oakley does not however suggest that the existence of a social relationship *necessarily* implies that it is beneficial. For example, marriage or other family relationships, while previously assumed to be inherently beneficial, have proven not always so and there are different effects for men and women. Relationships may even be harmful. Nevertheless there is evidence that lay support of pregnant women can have beneficial effects. Oakley's intention in this research was to examine the circumstances under which this might be so and the ways in which it works.

Midwives as providers of social support

According to Oakley (1992: 62):

> the professional ideology of midwifery emphasises caring for pregnant women on an individual basis as people enmeshed in social lives rather than merely vehicles for fetal growth, and midwives' focus on the presumed *normality* of childbirth also stresses the importance of *social care* as distinct from *clinical interventions*.

Therefore, she concludes, midwives are likely to provide social care and more likely to do so in the community. Oakley's attitude towards midwives in this study is contradictory since, despite these remarks, she later says that she considered using social researchers to provide social support in her study. This idea met with opposition from the Department of Health. If the study were successful it could imply that social scientists should be employed in antenatal clinics! Instead she decided that midwives were the obvious choice as researchers.

In her later description of the study, Oakley describes lengthy discussions with the research midwives appointed which encouraged them to avoid behaviour 'dictated by their midwifery training' (1992: 175). According to the women in the study it was not that the midwives were trained professionals which was important, but the midwives' own experiences as mothers (since all four research midwives had children of their own) that was the relevant factor. Apparently the study showed 'how the research role of the generalised social supporter can be preferred by women to the scrutiny of social workers and health visitors' (p. 185). So what did it tell us about *professional midwives*?

The definition of social support which Oakley 'wanted to operationalise centred on *listening*, to women, on *talking* to women about their pregnancy needs and circumstances and *giving information only when required*' (1992: 132). She stipulates that it was the 'personal relationships' between the research midwives and the women that was crucial and that 'social support was not clinical care, health education, or a device for raising the uptake of medical or other services' (p. 132), as normally understood by health professionals (including midwives).

There seems then to be a central paradox in the research design of this study. Though seeking to shed light on the meaning, processes and effects of social support, the study obscures what precisely the midwives' role might be. Oakley, in her conclusions reports on the view that the study was seen to reinforce the importance of *professional* support. Contradictorily she says if social support, as defined in the study, is effective it undermines the clinical standing and expertise of certain professional groups. By professional groups she refers only to obstetricians. What is not clear is whether she wants to argue that the midwives were effective social supporters because they were women or mothers or because they were trained, that is professional midwives. What is special about midwives' relationship with women? Could the same effects have occurred in Oakley's study if researchers were non-midwives as she seemed to imply earlier?

This seems to be a crucial point that fundamentally confuses the relevance or not of education and training for midwives and the value of lay, as distinct from professional, support. It also fails to analyse professional power (Hugman 1991). Oakley (1992: 327) collapses professional and general support together: 'the implication from the SSPO [Social Support and Pregnancy Outcome] study and others like it is that supportive care in pregnancy is best provided by women to women. The reason is not the biology of sex but the culture of gender, and the differences in professional training between midwives on the one hand and obstetricians on the other'. The assumption here is that the culture of gender intersects with the professional training of midwives. The difficulty with Oakley's analysis is that she does not examine the differences between midwives and those women they support. She does not explain under what conditions certain relationships may be supportive and others may not. When are social relationships unsupportive or unhealthy? Presumably it cannot be assumed that all midwife-client relationships will necessarily be supportive yet this seems to be exactly where Oakley's conclusions lead. A consideration of the literature on 'caring' seems useful here.

Moral identities

The division between men's work and women's work is, as I have indicated, a product of the social organization of the world of employment and the separation of the public and private spheres of human life. Traditionally women have been expected to undertake both unpaid care in the home and low paid caring work in the health service. Psychological explanations for this have suggested that a woman's identity is produced through this caring work. Drawing on object-relations theory, a woman's connection to others and sense of responsibility and concern for others constructs her identity. Suggestions that midwives, because they are women, are better equipped to care for other women have the effect of *essentializing* women. The implication is that what midwives do is a natural extension of being a woman. This is contentious for it takes the products (caring work) of social and political processes and *naturalizes* them.

In Chapter 2 we saw how midwives, in relation to doctors, take up a position of 'otherness' and claim an identity and role for themselves that is distinct from doctors. Midwives claim to 'care' for women rather than 'cure' them. In the same move they identify similarities between themselves and the women in their care – i.e. they are *women*. Such a claim glosses over differences between themselves and their patients. By claiming to speak for women, midwives assimilate women's needs into their own interests. Importantly, the ability of midwives to adopt this standpoint rests on their position of partial privilege in relation to 'other' women – that is, their professional power. This intensely political act by midwives at the same time mobilizes an 'ethic of care', a morality upon which their professional identity rests. Caring relationships, like other social relations, have a moral dimension.

Revaluing care

By turning to the work of moral philosophers such as Joan Tronto the importance of revaluing care as a central part of political life comes into view. This implies a revaluing of the caring work which women do and including them as full citizens in the public sphere. Tronto (1993) argues that women's morality is not about women and that arguments about the importance of care require a paradigm shift and a redrawing of moral boundaries. Although morality and politics are usually viewed as separate spheres, Tronto shows how they are 'deeply intertwined'. Morality is seen as what it is important to *do*, and refers to the conduct of relationships, while politics refers to decisions about the allocation of resources and maintaining public order. Women, in emphasizing the relational aspects of care, are deemed to be outside politics.

By drawing on aspects of daily life and emotion women's morality is, by definition, seen as secondary because the moral point of view is traditionally determined by reason, and justice is defined from the position of the autonomous, rational, disinterested individual. Finally, because women are consigned to the private sphere where caring work is done, they are ruled out of public life. Tronto, in mapping out these boundaries that characterize contemporary political thought argues that they need to be redrawn rather than abandoned. For her, 'the view that morality is gendered reinforces a number of existing moral boundaries and mitigates *against* change in our conception of politics, of morality and gender roles' (1993: 61, emphasis added). So, according to Tronto, feminist claims to a woman's morality as a strategy for including women in the public sphere are ineffective. On the contrary they reinforce the status quo.

Mendus (1993) also warns against emphasizing differences between men and women and advises caution in advancing an ethic of care which assumes that all women are (child)carers. Tronto (1993) maintains that the subordinate status of care (and carers) is not inherent in the nature of caring but results from current social values and moral boundaries. So rather than emphasizing differences between men and women, claiming that women are more moral, more able to care and nurture others, her view is that moral sympathy is not exclusively a woman's sphere. To suggest that it is merely reiterates the idea that men do not care, and that women as carers are outside the political sphere, marginal and without power.

Care and citizenship

Instead, by a closer examination of 'care', Tronto shows why all humans are interdependent, that autonomy and dependency are not simply binary categories. We are all more or less autonomous and dependent in different areas of our lives at different times. Accordingly, it is not simply that justice or democracy are greater goods or more important; rather, that a theory of care is embedded in notions of justice, and 'care as a practice can inform practices of democratic citizenship. If through the practices of giving and receiving care we were to become adept at caring I suggest that not only would we have become more caring and more moral people, but we would also have become better citizens in a democracy' (Tronto 1993: 167).

So caring should not simply be valued for its own sake (though it clearly is a moral good), but because it improves and strengthens democracy and is central to achieving justice. Revaluing care brings women into the public sphere and creates a more inclusive and effective democracy. 'Care is both a practice and a disposition' says Tronto (1993: 104). It is action that arises from a concern for others and recognition of their needs as articulated by them.

Mendus (1993) in contrast argues that an ethic of care is too narrow a concept and it is inappropriate to seek to extend familial relationships to political ones. Her criticisms of attempts to do so are based on the belief that care only relates to face-to-face relationships. When the concept of care is extended 'it can imply a loss of dignity for the recipient, and a convenient way of disguising the fact that he or she has claims in justice' (p. 23). For Mendus, receivers of care are demeaned when cared for by 'strangers' and instead there is greater dignity in claiming *rights*. Such a view does not of course revalue care or dependency but rather takes these as given. In essence Mendus wants to incorporate a feminist ethic which reveals that certain social roles and obligations which construct all human lives are contradictory.

Caring relationships and caring work as skilled work

In caring relationships exchanges of goods and services are frequently expected to be for love not money. Jennifer Mason (1994), in her discussion of kin and family relationships, suggests that we drop the dichotomy between labour and love which Graham (1983) argued was important for a feminist analysis of care. This earlier argument by Graham was that, in the case of women, the two aspects are frequently conflated and if women care about someone they are expected to care for them (Ackers and Abbott 1996).

Mason (1994) wants to propose that thinking and feeling are intimately connected, but that they are both 'activities'. For her, caring for someone does indeed involve the physical activities (labour/work) of shopping, cooking and cleaning, but her interest in thinking and feeling is to draw attention to the:

> *sentient activities* involved in shopping and cooking such as: noticing, interpreting and responding (not necessarily passively) to the needs of others, juggling dietary requirements and individual preferences, working these into some form of shopping plan often whilst shopping in relation to what provisioning choices are on offer, attempting to synchronise the timetables of family members in relation to eating, and orchestrating social relations around mealtimes.
>
> (Mason 1994: 10)

Drawing on DeVault (1991), Mason argues that these activities are commonly not recognized even by the person who performs them. Moreover they are skills. The focus on thinking and feeling as activities extends in Mason's analysis to the notion of *active sensibility*. This she suggests is feeling a responsibility is your own and acting accordingly. Mason then rejects any notion of 'emotion' as a fixed internal state. She also rejects the binary division between thinking and feeling of which other feminists are critical. For her 'emotional labour' encompasses aspects of both feelings for others and the skills of attending to those feelings. This she distinguishes from both labour and love in the context of specific family relationships.

Moreover, Mason's view is that such 'sentient activities' and skills are not necessarily transferable to other contexts. She believes it is not appropriate to universalize from this. We cannot assume that all women are better at caring than men or that men do, or do not, care. This implies that the abilities of midwives to care for women will depend on the specifics of individual relationships in a particular context. The implications for my discussion are therefore that midwives cannot necessarily claim that, by virtue of being women, they are caring or good at caring. Men too may care and there is an important sense in which men may legitimately become midwives.

Male midwives and men in the caring professions

Given the gendered processes that promote the caring activities of women and underplay their relevance to men, men may well have fewer opportunities to develop the skills of caring. The effect of sex-typing certain jobs is to problematize the men who take up such roles. How then may we view men in the caring professions and more specifically what should we make of male midwives?

I have already indicated that gender divisions at work may be seen as disadvantaging women as carers but does this have similar effects for men who do caring work? Men who do enter nursing have enjoyed higher paid and more senior jobs because even within the profession the skills and qualities attributed to men are more likely to secure them managerial positions. Men 'occupy managerial positions out of all proportion to their numbers in the caring professions as a whole' (Hugman 1991: 175) and now dominate the Royal College of Nursing (the professional association for nursing) (Littlewood 1991). Moreover, like men in other areas of employment, they are more likely to have uninterrupted employment without career breaks for childcare or unpaid domestic labour because they will benefit from a sexual division of labour at home.

For those who equate women and caring the notion of a male nurse or midwife is 'unnatural' (Hugman 1991) or 'a touchy topic' (Gaze 1987). Gendered identities dependent on certain notions of femininity and masculinity are mapped onto occupational identities of midwives and doctors. Men who do 'women's work' therefore are transgressing gender boundaries in ways that attract **homophobic** responses. Male midwives (like male nurses) are more likely to have questions raised about their sexuality and assigned the subordinate status of homosexual men within a hierarchy of masculinities. 'Hegemonic masculinity' (Hooper 1997) or what Hugman (1991) calls 'patriarchical masculinity' may be threatened by male midwives. Hence, these men are marginalized within the gender hierarchy by other men, but, in relation to women (both colleagues and clients) they are likely to maintain a relatively powerful position. There may be uncertainty over the relationship between men and caring but once chosen 'the career path is buttressed by other institutional sexisms' (Hugman 1991: 191).

In a study of male midwives Paul Lewis (1991) outlines the changes in legislation which permitted entry of men to midwifery from 1977 on an experimental basis, and on an unrestricted basis from 1983. This lifted restrictions on the training of men in midwifery which were enshrined in the 1975 Equal Opportunities legislation. Although such changes were supported by the Royal College of Midwives, few men were recruited to post-registration courses and few are being recruited to the newer pre-registration midwifery programmes (Kent *et al.* 1994). This may reflect the low numbers of men applying for midwifery, the attitudes towards male applicants in recruitment policies and practices of midwifery schools, and/or the wider negative attitudes to men becoming midwives. However, the findings of Lewis' study (himself a midwife) reveal interesting insights into the views of those men who do become midwives.

Compared to other studies of recruitment and retention in midwifery (Robinson 1986; Mander 1987) Lewis suggests that men entering midwifery are 'young, single, academically well-qualified and with a good background in nursing' (1991: 280). They were on average older than the women entering post-registration courses but only a third were married and one fifth were fathers. In noting this Lewis observes that marital status or having children had no effect on their careers (see above) and asked 'If the careers of men are not hampered by fatherhood, then why should careers of female midwives suffer as a consequence of motherhood?' (p. 280). This demonstrates a rather naive analysis of the gendered nature of work and the ways in which, as Hugman (1991) indicated above, 'other institutional sexisms' support the careers of men in the caring professions. Lewis also fails to acknowledge that women's relationship to domestic labour is different to their male midwifery colleagues. Moreover, in repudiating the idea that male midwives are more likely to occupy senior management positions (as in nursing) Lewis outlines the intentions of these men to pursue careers in clinical teaching and midwifery education which are also part of a promotional career ladder.

In describing the experiences of men in midwifery education and practice Lewis believes that they are generally well supported by colleagues and accepted by the majority of women receiving their services. Few described being rejected by women and in those cases it was usually religious and cultural practices that prohibited attendance by a man. Relationships with partners of labouring women were seen as particularly beneficial because the male midwives saw themselves as acting as 'role models' for new fathers and setting an example to men in general, showing that it is possible for men to be carers. Indeed because they were men they believed that they were more 'considerate and sensitive to a woman's wishes' (Lewis 1991: 282), unable to take for granted their ability to assess that woman's needs. This was contrasted with the position of a female midwife who, in their view could: 'identify with the woman's body, the pains of menstruation and the like [but] it doesn't mean she's going to gain the confidence of the woman if she doesn't conduct herself properly. Then she's just as likely to fail as a man' (Lewis 1991: 292). Thus, the men in this study emphasized features of the caring relationship as not contingent on sex differences but rather the approach to care and style of midwifery practice.

Gender relations were however important and male midwives recognized that some situations were more problematic than others. In particular the community setting presented difficulties for them compared to the hospital. Quoting one male midwife Lewis (1991: 290) tells us:

the only problem one might have in midwifery·is in the community. In postnatal care, one can break down the barriers surrounding
sexuality more easily in the hospital environment. Here people more
readily accept your role within an organised authoritarian situation,
regardless of sex. I think, however when you go into someone's home
and examine them on a bed on which they probably conceived, the
potential for embarrassment is going to be greater.

This implies that the ability of male midwives to assert themselves as
legitimate professional practitioners is related to the exercise of authority
and power in the hospital rather than a 'caring' approach.

In the community the relationship is seen as more ambiguous and
'caring' is more likely to be construed as a sexual encounter – that is, the
male midwife *caring about* the woman. Clearly interpretation of action is
indexically linked to the context and the removal of midwifery from the
public sphere of the hospital to the privacy of 'home' problematizes the
relationship in different ways. Of course in both settings gender relations
are constitutive of the encounter. But under the guise of professional
practice male power is concealed, whereas in the one-to-one relationship
in the home the clinical examination resembles more closely the intimacy
and gendering of sexual relations. I discuss more fully the organization of
sexuality in Chapter 7, and this will enable me to return to the issue of
male midwives again. Here though I suggest simply that arguments for
excluding men from midwifery are not supported in law or on ethical
grounds. At first sight there are however epistemological grounds for
disputing their legitimacy but these too begin to fall when we consider
extending those arguments to other midwifery relationships.

Acknowledging difference

There is an important sense in which men may not have experiential
knowledge that is relevant to being a midwife. That is, they are not themselves able to experience pregnancy and childbirth and interestingly this
was something that some of the male midwives in Lewis' (1991) study
regretted. However, such experiences are not prerequisites for becoming a
midwife even though some people might want to argue that they should
be. In suggesting that this important difference between men and women
is a basis on which men should not be midwives there is once again a
conflation of biological sex and gender.

By recognizing that gender, masculinity and femininity are social constructs, there is a space for men to assume other kinds of roles and responsibilities than are first dictated by '**hegemonic masculinity**' (see Chapter
7). Similarly, in so far as other midwives, despite not always being able to
gain experiential knowledge of what it is to be disabled, lesbian or black,
may be effective carers, then so too can male midwives be 'with women'.
Only if differences are seen as immutable and caring relationships contingent on similarities and shared experience can arguments against men
becoming midwives be supported. Such arguments are fundamentally
flawed in that they are not underpinned by an adequate theory of care.

If caring is understood as a reciprocal relationship of interdependence where differences between carer and cared for are part of that relationship, then the claim that in principle, all midwives (male and female) may care for all women may be substantiated. However, whether individual women receive care and support from individual midwives is contingent on a variety of other factors, not least the extent to which care is negotiated between them. It may still be the case that distortions of power and inequality structure that relationship in ways that neither party acknowledges, prohibiting fair and just negotiation, and it is for this reason that a sociological perspective on midwifery work is useful. In Chapter 9 I will examine the ways in which a more democratic approach to health care might be developed.

Conclusions

In this chapter I have examined theoretical explanations for the gendering of work. I have considered whether, and if so how, women are systematically disadvantaged at work. The concept of patriarchy was useful for outlining the ways in which men exercise power over women in the workplace, trade unions, professional associations, organizations and at home. While traditionally there has been a separation of the public and private spheres the position of women in the labour market or at work cannot simply be read off their domestic circumstances. Despite considerable differences between women, evidence shows that women usually occupy low paid, low status jobs. Much of the work they do is 'caring work' and sex-typing of jobs encourages women into jobs that are considered 'women's work'.

Midwifery may be seen as typically women's work. Historically it was an important part of the task of local, family and community-based women health practitioners. The medicalization of childbirth and growth of centralized maternity services weakened the ability of midwives to control their own practice. In the hospital midwifery work became routinized and fragmented. Increased specialization and a division of labour between obstetricians and midwives reinforced the work of midwives as subordinate.

Today midwives emphasize the 'emotional labour' they perform in caring for women. Students in training on new pre-registration midwifery education programmes claim that this is what makes midwifery distinctive. However, paradoxically this runs counter to other professional projects which present midwives as technically competent and well educated (see Chapter 3). Midwives may benefit from the deskilling of obstetricians if they remain a cheaper type of worker who can carry out similar work. Interprofessional relationships are being constrained and shaped by managerial strategies in today's health service. There is however, less indication that caring work or the traditional midwifery skills of listening to and supporting women will become more highly valued. This relates at least in part to the continuing tendency to marginalize care workers.

There is evidence that social support has beneficial effects on health in general and pregnancy outcomes in particular, yet this cannot overcome the deleterious effects of other social divisions and material deprivation.

Indeed the support that takes no account of such divisions is of limited value. While collectivist or communitarian principles of equality have emphasized rights to welfare as a fundamental part of citizenship, feminist ethics and theory points to a need to reframe the ways in which goods and services are distributed.

Philosophically, the links between an ethic of care and an ethic of justice must be more closely integrated. Suggestions that we feminize the state or that the caring professions adopt a woman's morality merely reinforce gender divisions and leave care as a marginal activity and carers excluded from political life. Instead I considered how, according to Tronto (1993), an ethic of care is central to a redrawing of moral boundaries and promoting a more effective democracy. Wider participation in public life, the promotion of better citizens and the development of more moral persons are seen here as requirements for a better society. In such a society midwifery may be seen not simply as 'women's work' but as a valuable and important way in which pregnant women are able to secure for themselves the health care they want.

In supporting the idea that men too may be effective midwives, I am not aiming to suggest that men should dominate midwifery work or that women should not be encouraged to choose a woman midwife if they prefer. But to play on gender divisions as a justification for excluding men from the profession has the effect, in the longer term, of weakening, rather than strengthening, women's position. By claiming midwifery is, or should be, 'women's work' is to reinforce gender divisions at work and to place care at the margins rather than at the centre of public life. Only when there is a willingness for everyone, including men, to see caring for others as part of their responsibility can we expect the material conditions for women (including midwives) to improve. An ethic of care needs to be seen as central to an ethic of justice. In the next chapter I examine more closely experiences of motherhood, fatherhood and caring in the home.

Summary

- This chapter examined the connections between knowledge, power and skill. The idea of midwifery as 'women's work' was explored.

- I have described the historical development of a division of labour in health care and occupational segregation in the NHS.

- Women do most of the caring work and the view that care comes naturally to women has undermined attempts to see this work as skilled. Caring work is generally low paid and of low status because it is done by women and because it is regarded as unskilled.

- Midwives and some feminist writers, in arguing for a revaluing of care, have continued to think in terms of a binary gender divide. A theory of care and an ethic of care that is central to justice and a part of citizenship is needed. Men too need to be seen as carers and caring. So while many midwives do provide the kind of care women want the idea that this is because midwives are women has a number of detrimental effects. I have suggested here that this perpetuates the view that women are naturally good carers and also undermines claims to skill and expertise. It also excludes men from midwifery.

- There are similarities between midwives and the women they care for but there are also important differences to be taken into account. Acknowledging these differences could help to clarify what constitutes the skills and knowledge of midwives and what counts as caring work.

Discussion points

- In what ways have women's ability to participate in the labour market been constrained?
- Is patriarchy a useful concept for explaining how work is gendered?
- What evidence is there for occupational segregation in the NHS?
- How are definitions of skill linked to gender?
- Are midwives and nurses likely to benefit from restructuring in the NHS?
- What does being 'with women' mean and how does the concept of care help us to understand what nurses and midwives do?
- What justification is there (if any) for excluding men from midwifery?

Further reading

Crompton, R. and Sanderson, K. (1990) *Gendered Jobs and Social Change.* London: Unwin Hyman.
Davies, C. (1995) *Gender and the Professional Predicament in Nursing.* Buckingham: Open University Press.
Tronto, J. (1993) *Moral Boundaries, A Political Argument for an Ethic of Care.* London: Routledge.
Walby, S. and Greenwell, J. with Mackay, L. and Soothill, K. (1994) *Medicine and Nursing.* London: Sage.

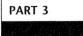

PART 3

CONSTRUCTING IDENTITIES

WOMEN AS MOTHERS

When asked about whether she wrote about her children in her poems, Adrienne Rich's explanation for not doing so was that 'for me poetry was where I lived as no-one's mother, where I existed as myself' (Rich 1995: 31).

Introduction

The discussion so far has highlighted the connections between knowledge, power and skill. In the last chapter, by examining ways in which skill is a gendered concept, I considered the reasons why caring work has been consistently undervalued. Gender, sexuality and the family were seen to structure the labour market. We saw that women do most of the caring work. In a liberal democracy, values of justice and autonomy have been assigned primary importance. The ethics of 'care' and reciprocity have been seen as of secondary importance and outside the public sphere of politics, instead confined to the private sphere of family and home. Women's relationship to work and the public sphere of politics has been marginal and contingent on their position within the family. The identity of 'woman' has been understood in terms of her reproductive capacity and ability to 'mother'.

In this chapter I shall explore the meaning of motherhood and women's experiences of mothering in the UK. Drawing on research that looks at mothers and motherhood my aim is to examine discourses of mothering and how these construct women's *identities* as mothers. I will then examine motherhood as a social institution and the position of women in relation to families. Finally I will consider the evidence of changing patterns of childbirth and suggestions that 'the family' is an increasingly contested form.

Twenty years since Ann Oakley's classic study of first-time mothers (Oakley 1979) the academic debates about women's relationship to motherhood have moved on. However the extent to which mothers today face similar issues deserves consideration and careful analysis. My own experiences of becoming a mother in the 1970s, like those of Ann Oakley and the women she interviewed, were characterized by tiredness, isolation, repetitive and unrewarding housework and childcare. Subsequently, like her, I struggled to raise a family and to develop a career, first as a nurse and later as a sociologist. Sociological theory gave me a new perspective on my experiences, a chance to rethink why being a mother was (and is) so difficult and to understand some of the tensions of family life. Becoming a mother implies a new set of social relationships which, while traditionally associated with marriage and family, are complex and multidimensional.

The first section of this chapter examines ideologies of 'motherhood' and women's experiences of mothering. What counts as a 'good mother' and how do women see themselves as mothers? The views we have of mothers are seen here as historically and culturally produced. Attitudes to mothers and mothering vary and have changed over time. However, there is a continuing controversy about the extent to which becoming a mother is 'natural' and represents a state of fulfilment for women. In addition the tasks associated with mothering – that is, caring for children – have commonly been seen as the responsibility of mothers. The idea that becoming a mother is 'natural' for a woman has been linked to ideas that mothering is an instinctual process. In contrast, it has been suggested that women may be fulfilled in other ways and that becoming a mother does not necessarily lead to fulfilment. Moreover, mothering need not be seen as something which only women can (or should) do.

The second section critically analyses the links between motherhood, marriage and 'the family'. This leads to a discussion of the position of women in families today. Mothers live in a variety of circumstances but are still primarily responsible for caring for children. They do most of the unpaid domestic work, but many mothers also work outside the home. Mothers who are managing home and work face particular kinds of struggles that have been well documented by feminist writers. In addition, many mothers and their children live in poverty and their circumstances relate directly to 'family policies'. The concept of 'family' will be seen as structuring health and welfare policies and affecting the health of these mothers and children.

The last section considers the evidence for changes in family forms. This will enable me to consider how far policies directed towards the family, mother and child health, maternity and welfare services take account of the diverse experiences of women as mothers. The view taken here is that we need a broad understanding of how women live and why being a woman need not necessarily be tied to being a mother. For some women who are mothers, their identities as both 'woman' and 'mother' are interlinked. Recognizing this does not mean that health care practices should be directed towards all women becoming mothers.

Ideologies of motherhood

There is an important sense in which 'mothers' and 'motherhood' have been invented. As Dally (1982) demonstrates, what it means to become a mother, theories and practices of mothering are historical and socially contingent. While there have always been some women who have become pregnant, given birth and produced a child, the ways they have done this have changed over time and vary across cultures. In 'modern' societies, pregnancy, as I have argued already in Chapter 2, became increasingly regarded as 'pathological', requiring medical intervention and management. Views and beliefs about women's bodies changed and the increased importance attached to scientific methods and knowledge was closely linked to the regulation and disciplining of women's sexuality and behaviour. Sex and reproduction were tied together and, as I shall discuss in Chapter 6, the common expectation was, and largely still is, that women will become mothers.

Becoming a mother is, even today, believed to mark the fulfilment of adult status for women. Even those women who are not mothers are often defined in relation to them, as potential mothers, childless, child-free or infertile. A woman's reproductive status is seen as central to her identity as a woman, a view that is *ideological* (Dally 1982; Phoenix *et al.* 1991). The lives of women are constrained and shaped by the idea that all 'normal' women become mothers and those who do not are believed to lead unfulfilled and unsatisfactory lives. The basic premise is that the essential 'real' woman is a mother. How women experience becoming a mother and mothering draws on discourses of mothering, representations of motherhood and systems of meaning. 'Mother' as *identity* and *practice* is constructed within a complex set of social relationships structured by power and inequality.

Representing motherhood

Images of pregnancy and childbirth (see Chapter 8) construct the pregnant woman as made whole, as complete, as a vessel or as incubator for the baby (see also Chapter 7). In medical and health care practice women are constructed as objects to be looked at and acted upon. Such practices and ideologies have been strongly resisted by feminists and birth activists who have sought to assert **agency** and **autonomy** for women. As we saw in the discussion of competing approaches to childbirth, advocating choice for women and greater control over their own bodies challenges the objectification of women and medical control (see Chapter 2). In Chapter 7 the debate over new reproductive technologies is frequently understood in terms of a struggle for control and recognition of women as *subjects*. Yet at the same time, some critics argue that **pronatalism**, the belief that women *should* become mothers, underpins these technologies, reinforcing a view that the identity of 'woman' is inevitably and irretrievably linked to the identity of 'mother'.

Cultural representations of mothers in art, popular culture and childcare or parenting manuals frequently idealize motherhood (Marshall 1991; Woodward 1997). Prescriptions about what 'good mothers' do and how mothers should behave provide a framework for evaluating the behaviour of women as mothers, and by extension, those women who are not mothers. The role of 'experts' in developmental psychology and childcare has been central to this process (Phoenix and Woollett 1991). However, recent studies of motherhood suggest that women's experiences of mothering are problematic and that there are negative aspects to being a mother. Importantly, becoming a mother is marked by a *loss of identity*, a loss of individuality associated with the expectation that the child comes first and the woman's needs are subordinate to it (Richardson 1993a). Richardson lists a number of losses associated with becoming a mother:

- loss of status;
- loss of identity;
- loss of independence;
- loss of privacy;
- loss of social networks;
- loss of an idealized and romanticized view of motherhood.

Motherhood then may be seen as a contradictory state, a paradox. In becoming a mother a woman is thought to become fully herself, fully realized as a woman by caring for others (especially children) and the subjugation of her interests and needs to theirs.

Motherhood and modernity

Caring for others is characteristically what defines 'woman' as 'mother' and, as I discussed in the last chapter, underpins ideas about what counts as 'women's work'. To become a mother is often thought to be associated with becoming selfless. Those women who are voluntarily child-free, who choose not to become mothers and articulate that choice are frequently therefore defined as selfish and uncaring. In her account of the 'modern mother' Benn (1998) suggests that in the 1990s things have changed for mothers; that in certain respects life has got better and in other ways much more complicated. Before examining these changes we need to understand the historical development of mothering in **modernity** and how motherhood has been characterized and criticized.

In much of the discussion of motherhood since the 1960s and 1970s feminists have been critical of the ways in which 'mothers' have been marginalized. This marginalization relates primarily to the exclusion of mothers, and by extension women, from public life and their relegation to the private sphere of the home. The separation of the public and private is part of the liberal tradition that in turn adopted patriarchal values. Men were viewed as independent, autonomous individuals, rational beings encouraged and able to participate in public affairs. In contrast, women – whose primary role was defined as reproduction – were seen as dependent, generalized (m)others. These gender differences, as I discuss below, were explained in terms of biological sex differences – women's 'natural' ability to have children and to care for them. So the experiences of women as mothers are historically produced and directly related to the development of 'modern society'.

The separation of the public and private spheres of life has been an important division that demarcated men from women and constructed their different experiences of social life. Men enjoyed the privileges of social status according to their occupation, class, ethnicity and sexuality (see Chapter 6) while women were relatively underprivileged and socially deprived. Traditionally a woman's status was tied to her husband's and, as we shall see, single or unmarried women were the least valued. Early feminists therefore focused their efforts on obtaining equal opportunities for women; on claiming a right to vote, to education and to jobs. These claims did not deny gender difference but argued for difference and equality (Richardson 1993a). Public policy drew on widely-held views about women as mothers and was directed towards ensuring that a woman's place was in the home. In political terms then, mothers had no public status and were not full citizens or subjects. Instead their role was to care for and respond to the needs of children (and men).

Mothers as carers

In the twentieth century childcare 'experts' have frequently been men whose 'emerging scientific interest in childhood also devalued women's own knowledge of infant care' (Richardson 1993a: 31). Though not engaged in childcare themselves these men felt able to tell women how to bring up children. Like pregnancy and childbirth, childcare became re-defined as an area for professional expertise and intervention. Medical men, psychologists and psychoanalysts such as Sigmund Freud, Frederick Truby King, John Bowlby, Donald Winnicot and Benjamin Spock led the field (Richardson 1993a). '**Maternal bonding**' and '**maternal deprivation**' were concepts that tied mothers to their children. These theories of child development and childcare have underpinned welfare and social policies since the 1950s. Mothering was thought to be something that came naturally to women and was expected to provide the means of personal satisfaction for them.

Analysis of childrearing manuals and theories of child development defined the role of mothers according to the wisdom of the day (Dally 1982; Richardson 1993a). The psychological health of children was seen as contingent on good mothering and although maternal deprivation, a concept first introduced by Bowlby in the 1950s, became increasingly controversial it (mis)informed public opinion and welfare policies for many years. According to Bowlby, separation of the child from its mother was a crucial developmental stage and for very young children was potentially damaging. The mental health of the child depended on successful bonding with the mother and an intimate and continuous relationship with her. Disturbances in the mother-child relationship, in Bowlby's view, led to trauma, mental disorder and instability in later life (Tizard 1991). His ideas were influential in shaping attitudes towards mothers working in the post-war years. The 'good mother' was expected to devote herself to the care of her children in a monogamous, hetereosexual family. Thus, ideas about mothering were closely linked with the concept of 'the family' and women's position within it. This has been the focus of concern for policy makers and feminists, though for different reasons.

Theories of mothering have continued to be important in shaping social policies and women's own views of motherhood. The 'modern mother' was encouraged to take heed of the 'experts' (Marshall 1991). Using a discourse analytic approach, Marshall identifies a number of key **accounting practices** in some of the more recent childcare and parenting manuals published in the 1980s (see Box 5.1). From this research we see that there is still considerable emphasis on the mother's responsibilities in childcare. Marshall highlights the contradictions that run through these manuals. She says, for example, that ideas that maternal love is 'natural', and common sense useful, contradict the view that mothers should consult experts and learn what is best for their child. According to Marshall, moral prescriptions and normative social values permeate this literature. I want to explore two key ideas in more detail here. First, the idea that **maternal instinct** has a part to play in explaining what motherhood means and what mothers do. Second, the view that mothering is *learnt*.

Instincts and culture

The 'maternal instinct' has been seen as part of the explanation for women's ability and willingness to care for others. This notion of 'instinct' natural-izes maternity, sees mothering as a natural process and, though it has

> **Box 5.1 A summary of Harriet Marshall's (1991) research looking at accounting practices in childcare and parenting manuals**
>
> Accounts of mothers, their roles and responsibilities included the following central ideas:
>
> 1 Motherhood as ultimate fulfilment – motherhood is exciting, joyful, pleasurable and rewarding. A positive experience.
> 2 Mother love is natural – there is a special relationship between mother and child characterized by maternal love.
> 3 Depression after childbirth is 'unnatural', an illness requiring expert help. 'Baby blues' are common and natural. Negative feelings about motherhood are unnatural and these women are 'ill'.
> 4 Good mothers are: flexible, use common sense but also seek *expert* knowledge and help which, based on observation, is more reliable than other women's experience.
> 5 It is *natural* for mothers to love their children but this is not enough to be a good mother. Expert advice and guidance is also necessary.
> 6 Good mothers operate most effectively in happy *families*, that is a nuclear family: mother, child and father. Single parenting is problematic and abnormal. Good mothers are also good wives and make sure that fathers play their part.
> 7 A mother's interests and needs are merged with her child's since she is seen as biologically adapted to meeting her child's needs.
> 8 Mothers must unselfishly share childcare with their partners (husbands) so fathers are involved and included. At the same time the limitations on fathers' involvement must be recognized since they commonly work and are prevented from being equal partners in childcare.
> 9 The ideal mother must be active in stimulating her child and provide a safe and secure emotional environment for 'normal' child development. Early deprivation is assumed to have long-lasting effects.
> 10 Social ills can be blamed on individual bad mothers.

been brought into disrepute by much feminist research, continues to influence contemporary attitudes towards women and mothering. In a discussion of 'the universal experience of motherhood' Kitzinger says:

> Birth is not just a matter of biology and primordial urges, but of cultural values. We have seen that in many societies the birth of a child is the consummation of marriage, rather than sexual intercourse, and that a girl does not achieve adult status until she has given birth. A baby has a profound effect on the relationship between a couple, and between them and other family members. The woman's identity changes too: *she becomes a different kind of person – a mother.*
>
> (Kitzinger 1992: 91, my emphasis)

So what is 'universal' about the experience of motherhood? How and why is the birth of a child linked to the adult status of a woman, marriage and family? In what sense can we talk of a woman's identity changing and her becoming a different kind of person?

Considered to be one of the most famous and influential 'experts' on female sexuality and childbirth, Kitzinger recognizes the importance of *culture* in shaping the experience of motherhood. However, contradictorily her celebration of 'motherhood' appears to cling to a notion of maternal *instinct* that is cross-cultural, universal and 'primordial'. She says 'human birth is a cultural act' and 'childbirth is never simply "natural"', and describes the myths, rituals and beliefs surrounding pregnancy and childbirth in different cultures (Kitzinger 1992: 91–2). Her vivid and absorbing accounts of the different birth practices in Sri Lanka, East Africa, New Zealand, the eastern Mediterranean, western countries and elsewhere highlight how 'culture' shapes experiences of birth. For example, birth is traditionally 'a female social space' and fathers and men are commonly restricted in how they participate in childbirth. 'In all societies men who have engaged in midwifery have done so at their peril' (Kitzinger 1992: 95), and, as I discussed in the last chapter, midwifery has traditionally been regarded as 'women's work'.

Kitzinger's anthropological work is valuable for highlighting cultural differences, for showing how childbirth experiences and motherhood are embedded in cultural values, beliefs and practices. It shows how conventions and traditions in our own society are historical and culturally specific. The discussion in Chapter 2 of how, in western societies, pregnancy and childbirth have been 'medicalized' demonstrates this. But what does it mean to become a mother and to what extent are mothers 'different kinds of persons' as Kitzinger suggests? What kinds of persons are mothers and what is the connection between being a woman and being a mother? The difficulty with Kitzinger's approach is that her study of 'culture' seems to leave untouched her notion of 'women' and 'mothers'. Though describing cultural difference she adopts a normative and pronatalist ideology towards women as mothers. Uncritically she reports 'traditionally the woman's most important role has been that of passing on culture through mothering' (Kitzinger 1992: 26). By championing the cause of mothers and valuing what mothers do, she appears to undermine and undervalue those women who are not mothers.

Learning to care

Kitzinger, while suggesting that mothers need to learn to care for a child, contradictorily appears to cling to the idea of maternal instincts. In the opening statement of her book *Ourselves As Mothers* she says 'birth is a biological process. Powerful physiological forces sweep a woman through the experience, and many things she does feel purely *instinctive*' (Kitzinger 1992: 1, my emphasis). Recognizing that 'culture' plays a part, she says that mothering is learnt in response to the needs of the child but that 'the second intensive learning phase is triggered by pregnancy, birth and the presence of the newborn young and the mother's interaction with them'

(p. 159). Although Kitzinger believes that motherhood has been idealized and romanticized, she does seem to essentialize women and see them all as potential mothers.

The idea that pregnancy automatically triggers a maternal response implies that women do have a maternal instinct, a view that many women expressed in Oakley's study (1979). So at the same time as seeing cultural norms as important in shaping experiences of childbirth and motherhood Kitzinger believes in 'the universal experience of motherhood'. In her view, the universality of motherhood seems to return to a biological or maternal instinct just at the point when 'culture' takes effect. It is not at all clear from her discussion just what might be instinctual and where, or how, culture plays a part. In her discussion of learning to care she says: 'at the beginning of life the human baby's appearance and behaviour provide very effective signals for the mother which stimulate her caring reaction to the child. The rounded shape of a newborn baby's head, the short face and large forehead, plump cheeks . . . are all evocative signals for maternal attention (Kitzinger 1992: 159).

We might conclude that both instincts and culture are important but rather than helping us to understand how they may interact Kitzinger leaves us with some notion of a universal experience of motherhood that appears to obscure the effects of culture.

Mothers as autonomous subjects

Everingham (1994), drawing on earlier feminist work, examines ideas about mothering and their political significance. She challenges the idea that mothering is simply a learning process helped along by 'maternal instinct' where 'all the mother must do is recognize what the objective requirements of the child are then meet these in socially prescribed ways' (1994: 7). Instead she argues for a view of mothering as 'an interpretative and potentially critical act' (p. 7) which implies a rethinking of the nurturing activity and a reformulation of 'autonomy' as a *relational* concept.

Everingham's argument is that mothering produces subjectivity, with both the mother and the child as subject. Rather than seeing autonomy and agency in developmental terms (an achievement of adult status) and expressed primarily in the public sphere, as is conventional in liberal theory, Everingham brings the *agency* of mothers into view. She says it is mothers who are 'creators of cultural meanings and human value systems' (1994: 7) who are active rather than simply responsive and are therefore fundamentally rational beings. This contrasts with Kitzinger's view that mothers merely transmit culture.

Everingham's aim is both to revalue nurturing activity, to see it as central to social life, and to undermine the split between the public and the private. In doing this she asserts that (women as) mothers are not generalized others, providing the environment for the development of the autonomous (masculine) individual. Instead they are subjects in their own right and are able to assert their own needs and interests during childrearing. Such a view fundamentally challenges the idea that mothers are passive or simply responding to the needs of others. It also suggests a need to rethink the work mothers do and reassess their role within, and outside, 'the family'.

Women and families

In the minds of many people having a baby is equated with the formation of a family. The stereotypical family is a mother, father and two children but it is a **stereotype**. It has been increasingly recognized, at least within academic discourse, that such a stereotype tells us very little about the lives of women, children and men today. But 'the family' as an ideological concept continues to influence policy and shape public opinion about a range of social issues.

The 'family' has historical roots in the rise of the white middle classes and increased dependency on wage labour since industrialization (Gittins 1985). As indicated in Chapter 4 a sexual division of labour between men and women and separation of 'work' and 'home' meant women, especially mothers, became financially dependent on men. The marriage contract secured property relations between men and women and ensured that inheritance rights were legitimated and motherhood was legalized (Smart 1996).

Mothers and marriage

Families in nineteenth-century industrial society were continuous with the past when small households were characteristic rather than, as popularly believed, large extended families with several generations or relatives living together. The high mortality rates associated with high birth rates meant that households comprised mainly two generations (Gittins 1985). The number of pregnancies and children born to women was higher but fewer children survived to adulthood. However, the differences between working-class and middle-class families were marked.

Middle-class women enjoyed better health and more assistance with childcare (nannies and servants). In contrast, in working-class families women often worked and looked after the children. Whereas marriage, for a white, middle-class woman, usually meant she was expected to stay at home and rely on her husband's income, this was less likely to be possible for her working-class sister. Gittins (1985) therefore argued that 'the family' is a class concept, which supported the patriarchal authority of middle-class men who kept their wives at home. A sign of success was being a family man with a wife and children at home provided for by him. Importantly, then, 'the family' represented a set of economic and social relationships between men, women and children. Marriage was also considered healthy for women whose sexuality was defined in relation to men (see Chapter 6).

The family or **familialism**, says Gittins, reflected middle-class morality and values of patriarchy, and the rule of the father was a central concept.

It was a model increasingly imposed on working-class families so that by the end of the nineteenth century the moral norm for married women, and especially those with children, was not to work. Although many working-class mothers did have paid work it tended to be intermittent and part-time. Traditionally the function and purpose of the family was to reproduce and women as mothers were expected to fulfil their function by reproducing labour power through childrearing and caring for the husband and father. The different roles of 'mothers' and 'fathers' constructed their identities as distinct from each other. More recently however, feminist analysis has been critical of both Marxist and functionalist approaches to the family and role theory. This has led to a reassessment of the significance and meaning of 'the family'.

Feminist critiques of the family

It can no longer be taken for granted that women, or indeed mothers, should be primarily engaged in childcare. As outlined above, early theories of childcare took as unproblematic the concept of the family and supported a division of labour between mothers and fathers. As I have suggested already, this idea has come increasingly under attack from feminist writers since the 1960s, but the legacy of these ideas remains (Richardson 1993a).

There are at least two strands in the feminist literature on mothering, one that celebrates mothering and the other which sees it as problematic. Some writers distinguish between mothering as a potentially fulfilling and transformative experience and the oppression of motherhood as a social institution (Segal 1995). In her discussion of the family Segal explains how the work of Rich (1995), Chodorow (1978), Ruddick (1982) and Gilligan (1982) supported ideas of maternal thinking and feminine subjectivity. Mothering could be rewarding and something to be celebrated. Segal says that for many women, especially in the USA, these ideas were inspiring and taken as valuing what mothers did.

According to other writers (e.g. Richardson 1993a), the reality of women's experiences of motherhood is that it is often isolating, unrewarding, repetitive and demanding. Oakley (1979) argued that women in her study found childcare rewarding but other aspects of housework, and the conditions under which it was done, unpleasant. These accounts highlight the oppression of mothers and the negative aspects of mothering. It is the institution of motherhood and women's position in the family that is seen as problematic. Constrained by beliefs about what a good mother is, women often describe feelings of guilt and frustration at their inability to find satisfaction in the role of mother.

Feminists have also challenged universal conceptions of mothering (Nakano Glenn et al. 1994). Marriage and motherhood are, in their view, not so beneficial to women and may even be bad for their health. Campaigns for birth control, abortion, greater reproductive rights for women as well as improved maternity care drew on these discourses, challenging the conventional belief that women should become mothers and conform to dominant ideologies of motherhood (see Chapter 7).

Despite more than 20 years of debate about the merits of (full-time) childcare by mothers and growing emphasis on 'shared parenting', childcare remains a contentious issue. There is no agreement about what counts as shared parenting or whether men should be encouraged to take on roles and responsibilities which some women have found rewarding (Edley and Wetherell 1995). The concept of 'the family' has come under wider scrutiny and debate. Psychoanalytic accounts of the family have been revised (Wetherell 1995) and feminists have shown that gender relations continue to be central to social life (and that heterosexuality is deeply problematic). Today it seems mothering is characterized by ambivalence. Ambivalence that may be seen as both a positive and creative force, and a negative, destructive one (Wetherell 1995; Parker 1997). Mothers are thought to both love and hate their children and mothering is experienced frequently as both intensely pleasurable and frustrating.

The role of fathers has been revisited with increasing suggestions that they too may 'mother' or at least share in childcare and be a positive force in the lives of children. It seems that men may, and should, 'care' and that traditional forms of masculinity should be reassessed (see Chapter 6). Yet research shows that men still undertake comparatively little childcare (Lewis and O'Brien 1987; Segal 1990, 1995; Richardson 1993a) and, in the UK particularly, public provision of childcare facilities has a record for being inadequate though this may be changing (Burgess and Ruxton 1996). This evidence suggests that, at least in the minds of policy makers and employers, until very recently, 'mothers' have still been expected to bear the burden of childcare. If women can afford to pay for childcare, and it is available, they may choose this option. But this remains an option only for a minority.

Working mothers

A significant number of mothers do paid work outside the home. However, the opportunities for women to combine a well-paid job with being a mother remain limited. There are women who are well-paid professionals and who may be able to afford to pay for childcare, enabling them to combine being a mother with working. But the majority of women, as we have seen, are in low paid, part-time and low status employment. Despite legislation in the 1970s to promote equal opportunities for women, the type of work women do and their experiences of work are distinct from those of men. This has been well documented by economists (Gardiner 1997; Hatt 1997) and sociologists (Dex 1988; Crompton and Sanderson 1990; Walby 1990) who explore the idea that women are 'secondary workers'. In Chapter 4 I discussed the ways in which work is gendered and how midwifery, and many other jobs women do, are seen as extensions to what women do naturally – that is, care for others. Theoretical explanations for these patterns in the labour market are closely linked to the position of women in families and their role as primary childcarers. Although mothers have often, in public policy, been expected to be engaged in childcare, the financial circumstances of many women means that paid employment is an important source of income for them.

In a recent study, Hewison and Dowswell (1994) note that in the UK fathers of children under 5 work the longest hours in Europe. The numbers of mothers of under-5s who work is the second lowest in Europe and the third lowest for mothers of children aged 5 to 9. The ages of a woman's children are highly significant in influencing whether or not she is in paid employment. Men (fathers) continue to see themselves as 'the breadwinner' and mothers often work part-time. The jobs women do, especially mothers, are more likely to be part-time, lower paid and of lower status. As we have already seen both vertical and horizontal occupational segregation describes the hierarchical structuring between employment of men and women. While social attitudes continue to define women in terms of their potential or actual role as mothers, discrimination and disadvantage in the workplace will remain. Moreover women themselves may want part-time employment because it combines with childcare, while men are less able to take this option both because of the structure of the labour market and social attitudes.

The estimated cost of childbearing and childrearing for a mother of two children in the UK is more than half her potential *lifetime's* earnings (Joshi and Newell 1987 cited in Hewison and Dowswell 1994, my emphasis). After having children, a woman is likely to experience downward occupational mobility – a lower paid, lower status job or reduced career prospects. This may be because mothers change to lower paid or part-time jobs. It may also be because they find their promotion prospects reduced or because they are not geographically mobile due to either marriage or motherhood. According to Hewison and Dowswell (1994) most women appear to accept that childcare is their primary responsibility. Though the absence of public provision makes it difficult to see what alternatives are available to them, mothers do continue in work and some choose to, and are able to, progress their careers.

The experiences of working mothers and the effects of 'the double day' or 'the dual burden of work and home' are frequently described as a 'juggling act'. In their influential research, Brannen and Moss (1988, 1990) have documented the effects of women returning to work full-time after the birth of their first child and of those mothers in 'dual earner households' in the 1980s. They questioned the assumption that women returning to work was 'a bad thing' and explored how mothers managed their work and home lives. They highlight the management skills of mothers, enabling them to combine full-time work with shouldering the major responsibility for childcare and domestic work at the same time. In these heterosexual couples, men did very little housework and limited childcare, 'helping out' rather than taking an equal share. Normative assumptions about gender roles in the household continued to construct the division of labour and attitudes towards working mothers.

Health and work

The impact of working mothers on mother and child health has been, and continues to be, a matter of concern and controversy. It is not at all clear how far the benefits outweigh the costs (Doyal 1995). Having paid work provides some women with an important source of identity, companionship, higher social value and economic benefit. Improved economic circumstances will have a positive effect on health (see below) (Payne 1991). At the same time there is often stress and a physical burden associated with combining domestic work, including childcare, and paid work (Brannen and Moss 1990). In a review of research on the psychological health of women Hewison and Dowswell (1994) say that the relationship between these factors is complex and there are significant differences between women. Some types of work may be more or less beneficial for some women since there are differences between women (for example age, class and ethnicity) and women do different kinds of work (Doyal 1995). However, those *mothers* who do part-time paid work are considered to enjoy better health than those who do full-time paid work or those who do not do paid work at all.

Hewison and Dowswell (1994) were interested in how working mothers managed to care for a sick child as a measure of how they juggled home and work. They concluded that this juggling act was a solo one and that mothers, not fathers, bear the costs of their children's ill health. Working mothers, sometimes with the help of female relatives, provided care for their child while fathers contributed very little and employers virtually nothing, except 'sympathy' and agreement to changing shifts or holidays (a cost to the woman herself). Access to networks of social support, especially grandmothers are particularly important for (working) mothers caring for young children (Brannen and Moss 1990; Gardiner 1997). In addition, Hewison and Dowswell challenged generally held beliefs that working mothers are 'unreliable' workers. They argued that there are good economic and social reasons why public investment in childcare and supporting parents, especially mothers, is needed. Examples of more women-friendly family policies, which emphasize the responsibilities of the state in providing childcare, are available in Sweden and elsewhere in Europe and could be adopted in the UK (Millar 1996).

Marriage, motherhood and poverty

In many respects the financial security of women is circumscribed by their relationship to men. Historically, as we have seen, the concept of 'the family wage' was central to the claims made by working men for higher wages and better working conditions. Yet this assumed that men were indeed the breadwinners and that women were both married to men and were financially dependent on them. For many women this was the case even though not all men were able to earn a 'family wage'. At the same time arguments for a family wage effectively undermined the case for women who work to be paid a decent wage. Even today on average, men's wages are higher than women's. Many women are married and living in families but many live in diverse circumstances. There is therefore a need to carefully assess the extent to which mothers (and children) live in poverty both inside and outside (or after) marriage.

The statistics on poverty have been criticized for obscuring the circumstances of women, and for making women's poverty invisible (Pahl 1989;

Payne 1991; Glendinning and Millar 1992). Using 'families' or 'house-holds' as a unit of analysis says very little about how income is managed within those households, or the circumstances of individual members. A more careful analysis of how money is managed within marriages suggests that the redistribution of wealth or transfer of resources in 'families' is a complex matter (Pahl 1989; Payne 1991). Even in families women do not necessarily benefit from the wages of men in an equitable way. Power relations influence the distribution of resources and, within marriage and families, women generally lack power. This explains, at least in part, why women who have left violent or abusive relationships and other lone mothers felt 'better off' on their own with greater control over their finances (Pahl 1989; Groves 1992). However, access to well-paid employ-ment, or adequate benefits, is the primary means of avoiding poverty. This is difficult for women and the expectation that mothers are primary childcarers limits the opportunities open to them, as we have already seen.

Low pay and the costs of childcare

Women on average earn less than men even when they are doing com-parable jobs (see Chapter 4). Maternity pay and child benefit does not replace the loss of earnings and costs of childcare to which most mothers become liable (Joshi 1992). Even where a mother returns to her full-time job after maternity leave, the costs of childcare will most often be seen as being paid from her salary. The decisions mothers make in relation to taking up paid employment are frequently offset against the costs of childcare in a calculation that seldom plays a part in men's relationship to the labour market because a woman's wage is usually seen as secondary.

Many mothers who are employed work part-time in low paid jobs. Low pay increases the chances of poverty and creates a poverty trap for those who cannot earn enough to cover the costs of childcare. Mothers (especi-ally lone mothers) are therefore more likely to have to rely on a combina-tion of low pay and benefits such as family credit, and need assistance with childcare (Bryson et al. 1997). As well as being gendered, poverty is shaped by other social divisions such as class, ethnicity and disability. Therefore mothers from diverse social groups will suffer to a greater extent compared to others. Working-class girls are more likely to see mother-hood as affording them adult status and may therefore be trained to be low paid women (Buswell 1992). Racism will affect the opportunities open to black women (Cook and Watt 1992) while other religious and cultural norms may also influence attitudes to mothers working.

Another consequence of low pay and a work record interrupted by periods of childcare is that mothers' contributions to pension schemes, and those of the employer and the state, are affected. They are therefore likely to be living in poverty during old age (Groves 1992; Ackers and Abbott 1996). A woman's access to pension rights has been dependent on her husband's contributions. Where women contribute to occupational schemes themselves the benefits of an occupational pension, even for better-off women in pensionable employment, compares unfavourably with male contemporaries. Common life events such as becoming a mother, divorce, remarriage or widowhood all have detrimental effects on the pensions of women in ways which are distinct from the life chances of men. 'Women's greater share of unpaid domestic work and their labour market position, including low pay, have inhibited their ability to generate an adequate income for old age' (Groves 1992: 205). Women who are mothers are particularly disadvantaged in this respect.

Poverty, mother and child health

A major impact of poverty is on the health of mothers and children and on pregnancy outcomes (see Chapter 2). Differences between women are important for explaining how they experience poverty. 'While poverty disproportionately affects Black families, studies which address women's experiences of poverty focus disproportionately on white families' (Graham 1992: 211). Drawing on a range of data, Graham says that black women are more often employed in low paid jobs and are more likely to live in households with children. In addition, racism affects their chances of accessing social security benefits to which they are entitled. There are also differences between the extent to which black and white mothers are allowed (by their partners) to manage household income. While often neither have control over the money available to them, they do spend a considerable amount of time and effort 'making ends meet', 'managing' or 'just surviving'. Graham's study and other research shows that many mothers in low income households have difficulty in affording basic necessities because the level of income is so low and after paying the bills there is little left for food. Food and adequate nutrition is a basic requirement for good health. Where food is limited mothers put their own needs last, giving what is available to their male partners and children first. In order to limit their use of fuel some mothers only have the heating on when children are at home. Mothers try to protect the health of their children at costs to themselves.

Although women, as a group, live longer than men they have poorer health during their lives (Payne 1991). The complexities of measuring health and poverty are beyond the scope of this chapter but what is evident from the literature and from the statistics available is that the effects of gender are often ignored. Feminist critics of social policy such as Payne, and Glendinning and Millar (1992), do however provide substantial support for the argument that poverty and health inequalities are gendered. Women as mothers, especially of young children, are particularly vulnerable to the effects of social deprivation (such as poor quality housing, low incomes) and, associated with this, poor health. Those who are full-time childcarers and unpaid domestic workers with no paid employment 'report higher levels of chronic illness and poorer health overall' (Payne 1991: 128).

Nineties 'New Man'

Traditionally the social relationship of father has been as 'provider' of financial support. Caring for children was essentially regarded as woman's work and this view was supported by discourses of motherhood. More recently, changes in the family have been associated with a crisis of masculinity and the role of fathers is being critically reassessed. A growing emphasis on fathers' rights and responsibilities has emerged during the 1990s.

Feminist criticism of the position of women in the family and their subordination to the needs and demands of men and children drew attention to the non-participation of fathers in most aspects of childcare and domestic labour. Increasingly fathers were being challenged to take on more responsibility at home and to become more involved in caring for children. Studies of families and fatherhood indicate that changes in fathering practices are more complex than this earlier characterization suggests, but that the father as 'breadwinner' model continues to dominate contemporary family life in the USA (e.g. Lewis 1987; Pleck 1987; Marsiglio 1995a), and the UK (Edley and Wetherell 1995).

Men, it seems, are sometimes willing to take on more of the caring tasks but are also sometimes unable to because of the demands of paid employment. Others choose not to get involved perhaps because they feel unskilled in caring (Lupton and Barclay 1997). However, Segal (1990) suggests that the pace of change is slow, and that although attitudes to fathering, and experiences of fathering, may have altered the actual amount of work done by fathers in the home has changed very little. Moreover she reports that studies in the 1980s showed that men chose which tasks they did (usually certain aspects of childcare but little housework) and left the rest to their partners. She concludes:

> men's resistance to change, however, not only reflects real economic and social pressures, and both sexes' attempts to shore up a man's sense of self-esteem around a traditional masculinity; it also enables men to remain cushioned and privileged in relation to women. It is simply not in men's interest to change too much, unless women force them too.
>
> (Segal 1990: 41)

Those men who do become more involved in shared parenting are evidently less committed to gender roles and more likely to be viewed as 'in touch with their feminine side'. This view suggests a breaking down and transformation of gender identities and a more complex relationship between 'masculinities' and 'femininities' (see Chapter 6). So, reconstructing fatherhood is linked to a deconstruction of masculinity and recognition that macho male power is less valued than previously, at least in certain contexts. This does not however necessarily imply a dramatic shift in gender power relations, rather the growing attention given to fathers and fathering may be at the expense of power for women to control their own fertility and reproductive processes (Segal 1990; Callahan 1995). Fathers' rights are frequently presented in opposition to mothers' rights (Overall 1995; Shanley 1995) (see Chapter 7).

Gay men and 'the family'

In a discussion of 'pretended family relationships' Weeks (1991) describes the continuing and growing emphasis on family values in the 1980s. He argues that there has been a liberalization of attitudes towards sex. But, in the UK, the furore that developed around new legislation affecting local authorities' treatment of homosexuality indicated a conservatism in public opinion. Surveys of public attitudes showed that the majority rejected the idea of homosexuality as a lifestyle or as 'a pretended family relationship'. In 1987 strong opposition to the ability of both gay and lesbian couples to adopt children also indicated that the heterosexual 'family', or at least some version of it, was morally acceptable but that other arrangements were not (see Chapter 6). The continued marginalization of lone mothers also indicates that fathers, as heterosexual men, enjoy a valued social position, despite a growing recognition that it is more often heterosexual fathers who are perpetrators of sexual and child abuse and violence in the home (Weeks 1991; Maynard and Winn 1997). In contrast the opportunities for homosexual men to care for a child remain extremely limited.

Motherhood and changing family forms

In this final section I want to examine the claims that there is 'a crisis in the family' and the evidence for changing family forms. Those commentators who talk of 'a crisis' in family life are likely to put the family at the centre of social life believing that families are essential to maintain social order and the health of the nation. Yet the debate around the changing composition of households and diversity in family forms has attracted interest from a wide range of researchers and policy makers. In a study carried out for the Joseph Rowntree Foundation, Utting (1995) explains that concern about the welfare of children and family breakdown does not necessarily reflect traditional moral values but a recognition that economic and social deprivation impacts on families and affects the ability of adults to 'parent'. For the purposes of his study Utting redefines 'family' as 'dependent children with their principal adult carers' (Utting 1995: 9) and looks at the trends and transitions in demographic statistics (see Box 5.2).

There are a number of different types of two parent 'families' included in Utting's data. Two parent families may comprise:

- Children living in a two parent family with married parents who are both 'biological' parents.
- Children living in a two parent family where parents are not married though both are 'biological' parents.
- Children living in a two parent family where parents are married but are not both 'biological' parents.
- Children living in a two parent family where parents are not married and are not both 'biological' parents.

When interpreting population statistics Utting warns that reports of 'the imminent death of the "traditional" two parent family have . . . been grossly exaggerated' (1995: 11). Instead, using data from the General Household Surveys between 1971–92, he argues that eight out of ten households with dependent children are headed by two parents and in the majority of cases the child lives with his or her birth parents.

Box 5.2 Trends and transitions in demographic statistics

- Marriage rates have reached their lowest point since records began more than 150 years ago.
- Cohabitation has increased in a quarter of a century, from the experience of 6 per cent of brides before their wedding day to 60 per cent.
- Childbearing, like marriage, is being postponed. The average age at which women give birth to their first child has risen from 24.7 in 1961 to 27.7 years.
- Nearly 1 in 3 births (31 per cent) occur outside marriage, compared with 1 in 16 (6 per cent) 30 years ago.
- There are fewer large families and fertility rates have declined from a post-war peak of 2.9 children per woman in 1964 to 1.8.
- There has been a sixfold increase in the annual divorce rate since 1961. If current trends continue four out of ten new marriages will end in divorce.
- One in 5 families with dependent children (21 per cent) are headed by a lone parent compared with 1 in 12 (8 per cent) in 1971. The proportion of families headed by single mothers who have never been married has grown from 1 per cent to 7 per cent.
- One in 12 dependent children (8 per cent) are living in step-families. By age 16 about 6 per cent of children will have lived in married couple step-families and 7 per cent in cohabiting couple step-families.
- Two out of three mothers with dependent children either have jobs or are actively seeking work compared with fewer than half 20 years ago. Economic activity among mothers of children under 5 has increased from just over a quarter to almost half.
- Employment patterns over 15 years have become increasingly polarized between 'dual earner' families and homes where nobody has a paid job.

Source: Utting 1995: 7.

At the same time the number of lone parents is on the increase and one in five families are headed by a lone parent which is usually a mother (see Table 5.1) (though children may live in a lone parent family for only part of their childhood – see below). Some researchers believe that marital breakdown has a detrimental effect on the health of the nation and that men and children in particular suffer as a result (McAllister 1995). 'Marital problems' are, in their view, a frequent source of psychological ill health for women, especially those who are divorced. However McAllister's analysis interprets this data as meaning there are benefits to a 'good marriage'. It is equally plausible that tensions in the family and marital relations indicate good reasons for divorce. So while claiming not to advance a particular

Table 5.1 Household type 1971 and 1992

Household type	1971 %	1992 %
Two parent	92	79
Lone mother	7	19
single	1	7
widowed	2	1
divorced	2	6
separated	2	5
Lone father	1	2

Source: General Household Survey in Utting (1995).

moral position on marriage, McAllister's research does take as its starting point the view that marriage provides 'a healthy environment' and that divorce is bad for your health. These are controversial issues and competing interpretations draw on different values and beliefs about the position of women in families and the causes of marital stress.

Let us examine the implications of the statistics shown in Table 5.1 and what Utting and other researchers have to say about them.

Lone mothers

In the 1990s lone mothers were frequently the focus of political controversy (Pheonix 1996) and at the centre of debates about the 'New Labour' government policies to encourage them into work (Bryson *et al.* 1997). The numbers of lone mothers is on the increase (see Table 5.1 and Millar 1992) and, associated with this, the number of births outside marriage has also increased (these data are estimated using birth registration details) (Utting 1995). Lone mothers are frequently seen as representing a threat to the fabric of society, causing moral panic (Roseneil and Mann 1996) and social anxiety (McIntosh 1996).

The category 'lone mothers' may include those women who give birth outside marriage (never married), those who are divorced, separated or widowed (who may have given birth while married or become mothers during marriage). The majority of lone mothers are women who have been married. Their lone status is defined in terms of their relationship to a man (who may or may not be the father of their child). Clearly, changing attitudes towards marriage and the family have an influence on the numbers of women who may be counted as lone mothers. But it is not at all clear as to why these changes are occurring and different views of the data are expressed in the literature. For example, it could be that this trend marks a neglect of women by men or an active choice by women to mother alone (Bortoloaia Silva 1996). So have these women rejected marriage or are they victims of 'family breakdown'? Can lone mothers be 'good enough mothers' (Bortoloaia Silva 1996)? What are the implications of being a lone mother?

Analysis of the position of lone mothers relates to the kinds of questions one poses about them. As indicated already one of the major implications of being a lone mother, especially a mother of very young children, is the increased likelihood of living in poverty (Millar 1992). This can in turn be linked to lone mothers' exclusion from, and marginalization within, the labour market. Access to well-paid jobs for women will affect the opportunities available to those lone mothers who are seeking work. The availability of publicly funded childcare and social security payments for lone mothers both impact on their participation in paid employment (Bryson *et al.* 1997). The links between marriage, motherhood and employment may therefore be seen as intertwined. However, since some women choose not to have children, or to have children and not marry, these links may also be seen as having become loosened (Bortoloaia Silva 1996).

Lone mothers and the dependency culture

For many years lone mothers have been represented as a burden to society and as epitomizing the '**dependency culture**' because of a belief that there are high costs associated with supporting them. Millar (1992, 1996) explains that the 1991 Child Support Act signalled a significant change in policy. Millar says that in the UK the relationship between three potential sources of income for lone mothers – earnings, child maintenance and benefits – shifted. The state aimed to transfer the 'burden' to fathers who were expected to pay towards the costs of childrearing, and increasingly mothers have been 'encouraged' (or pressured) to return to work. This Act and the work of the Child Support Agency was controversial because it required lone mothers to name the father of their child and imposed penalties if they did not. At the same time it reinforced the view that women, especially mothers, should be dependent on men for support rather than rely on state support (Westwood 1996). Many women did not want maintenance from the father of their child or any contact with him and others had already agreed settlements with their ex-partners. Moreover, Millar (1992) argues that most women would not be better off as a result of these new policies.

According to Millar (1996) policies relating to the position of mothers are most important in determining the financial position of lone mothers. It is by virtue of being mothers rather than being lone mothers that they are relatively poor. In Millar's view (following Lewis 1992) it is the extent to which welfare policies reflect a view of the man as 'breadwinner' and how the breadwinner wage is replaced that is important for lone mothers. So normative assumptions about gender relations continue to shape public policy and the experience of lone motherhood is constructed according to whether claims for support rest on a definition of 'women as wives, mothers or workers' (Millar 1996: 112).

Moral decline

Other important disputes about lone motherhood include a resistance to the suggestion that lone mothers are the cause of moral decline and rising crime. The treatment of lone mothers at the hands of the media has been seen as part of an anti-feminist backlash against women who want to raise children on their own. This is one explanation also given for the growing attention to the role of fathers, as I indicate in Chapter 6 (Roseneil and Mann 1996). These discourses construct the lone mother as arrogantly choosing to mother on her own, rejecting marriage, fathers and the family. Yet the other side of this is the view that these women are victims of economic uncertainty, material deprivation and a patriarchal welfare state. Roseneil and Mann argue that such a polarization of the debate is unhelpful, for it mobilizes a set of dichotomies that do not match the experiences and lives of lone mothers (Morris 1992).

Cohabitating mothers

According to McRae (1993) there have always been informal marriage practices and the idea that cohabiting mothers today represent a decline in the wedded bliss of the 1950s is misleading. Post-war, the 1950s represented the peak of marriage which had increased since Victorian times and was associated with the growth of industrial capitalism and the development of social policies which shifted the financial burden of women and children onto men. Marriage represented the achievement of adult status and in McRae's view continues to be an attractive option for many women. But cohabitation has increased and the number of mothers in cohabiting relationships has risen (see also Dallos and Sapsford 1995). McRae's study, which defined cohabitation as 'a consensual union', estimated that 4 per cent of children live in cohabiting families, that the numbers are on the increase but that cohabiting *precedes* rather than *replaces* marriage. The focus of the study assumed cohabitation to refer to heterosexual relationships and the primary interest was in why women who are mothers continue in cohabiting relationships or 'will not marry' (McRae 1993: 107).

It has been suggested that cohabitation is little different from marriage. MacRae's view is that the rise in cohabitation does not ultimately represent a threat to marriage or 'families'. Instead cohabiting couples and their children may be seen as 'social marriages'. She concludes that 'fewer than 1 in 2 long-term cohabiting mothers will remain unmarried indefinitely' (McRae 1993: 105) and that those couples who lived together prior to marriage were more likely to separate within 15 years compared to married couples who did not. According to McRae, many cohabiting mothers eventually get married.

In McRae's study, for cohabiting mothers, pregnancy was itself often one of the principal reasons given for setting up home together though other factors played a part. Cohabitation is often, but not always, seen as a trial marriage – falling in love and the desire for a regular sexual partner were also given as reasons for cohabiting. Becoming pregnant was also a reason for not getting married but to delay marriage (unlike in the past). The high cost of a wedding and fear of divorce were also considered important reasons for not marrying. Cohabitation was more common prior to second marriages, often because one partner was still legally married to someone else.

Cohabitation and the law

McRae says that, for the mothers, legal ties between cohabiting partners and themselves, or between the cohabiting fathers and their children were not a priority. Instead mothers sometimes saw freedom from these as an advantage. McRae appears to reject this view because she concludes that cohabiting mothers are 'ignorant of the law' and public policy should enforce the private responsibilities of cohabiting 'family' members. She says cohabitees should be made aware of their legal position. Her moral stance is made explicit in the final remark that 'cohabiting couples who wish to avoid rights and obligations may be advised also to avoid having children' (McRae 1993: 107)! Cohabiting mothers, then, are seen as a target for public policy.

Diversity in family forms

That there is increased diversity in 'family forms' cannot be denied. The 'pattern of diversity' has increased with the numbers of cohabiting and step-families as well as lone parent families rising (Dallos and Sapsford 1995). However, the majority of children still live with their married, natural parents or with their cohabiting natural parents (Dallos and Sapsford 1995):

> Family life of the married-with-children variety (including couples at an earlier or later life stage, before or after the period of childcare) does seem to be a statistically very common domestic arrangement. It appears also to remain popular even with those who have tried it and decided to withdraw. Of the marriages existing at the beginning of 1987, one in eighty was broken by divorce before the end of the year; on the other hand in a third of all marriages contracted during 1987, one or both partners had previously been divorced.
>
> (Dallos and Sapsford 1995: 138)

These statistics suggest the appearance of stereotypical nuclear families, but beneath these there is diversity between ethnic groups and within 'families' (Dallos and Sapsford 1995). The ideology of 'the family' while continuing to shape public policy has been, and continues to be, questioned by researchers, individuals and some social groups (see Chapter 6 for a discussion of lesbian mothers, 'pretended family arrangements' and homosexuality). Yet discourses of 'the family' also continue to shape experiences of diverse family forms.

Anti-sexist living arrangements

In an interesting discussion of 'anti-sexist living arrangements', VanEvery (1995) provides an insight into how some women have attempted to resist adopting the traditional roles of wife and mother (see also Gordon 1990, 1994; Chandler 1991). VanEvery explores the negotiations and struggles between heterosexual women, their partners and members of collectives, to 'swap' or share domestic tasks and mothering and live in anti-sexist ways. This is seen as a struggle because of the normative effects of widespread attitudes to marriage, motherhood and families. In effect these women attempt to de-link the roles of 'wife, mother and worker' and redefine them in flexible ways. Yet wifely duties are not seen as wholly related to being married – even those who cohabit may adopt the role of 'wife'. Having children has a significant impact on how living arrangements are organized but, according to some of the women in this study, men may 'mother' and women may be defined primarily as workers.

The complexity of the different arrangements in these relationships points to the possibilities of alternatives but they are usually constructed in opposition to, and as a resistance to, familialism and ideologies of motherhood. The constraints on developing alternatives are apparent. Women have to rely on the willingness of male partners to renegotiate living arrangements. The effects of wider social attitudes towards men who mother or take care of the children, or women who raise children without men, shape their experiences and the 'success' of these alternatives. Lack of support for men who 'mother' was described by VanEvery (1995). Gender continues to be produced through these relationships and 'the division of housework is clearly affected by the gender of members of the living arrangements' (VanEvery 1995: 127). While gender differences could be 'overcome' or accommodated they continued to play a part. Men frequently remained uncommitted to an equal division of housework, even in cases where they took responsibility for childcare. So while the traditional family has been heavily criticized, these examples of cohabiting and collaborative living arrangements do present other models (see also Chandler 1991). But the extent to which they are distinct from stereotypical families in practice (as well as in law), or afford opportunities for anti-sexist living and childrearing remains an open question and a matter for daily struggle (e.g. Gordon 1990).

Age and motherhood

Birth statistics indicate that, in Britain, the average age for a woman having a first child is older than in the past and that the number of children a woman has is fewer than before (see Box 5.2). The reasons for these changes are complex but relate to the availability of contraception and abortion (see Chapter 6) and changing attitudes to becoming a mother. There is however evidence that many people think there is 'a right time' to have a baby. In their discussion of this idea Phoenix (1991a, 1991b) considers attitudes towards teenage pregnancy and Berryman discusses 'older motherhood' (Berryman 1991; Berryman and Windridge 1995; Berryman et al. 1995).

'Older motherhood' usually refers to women over the age of 35 who become pregnant and give birth. Berryman (1991) in a review of the literature on older mothers describes the medical perspective as emphasizing risk factors and pathologies associated with reduced fertility and an ageing maternal body. Emphasis is placed on beating 'the biological clock' and, from a medical point of view, delaying childbirth is ill-advised. In addition the belief that older mothers are usually women (particularly those who are first-time mothers) who have intentionally delayed having a baby in order to pursue a career is, according to Berryman, debatable. She argues that her study of older mothers (over 40 years old) indicates that these women are not 'career oriented', do not see their role as 'financial provider' and live in 'traditional types of family setting' (Berryman 1991: 115).

However in her later research with Windridge and with Thorpe (Berryman and Windridge 1995; Berryman *et al*. 1995) Berryman suggests that older mothers are likely to be of higher educational and occupational status, and more often pay for childcare. From a psychological perspective she also suggests that there are benefits to having a child later in life. Older mothers may be considered more 'mature' and 'better skilled' in parenting because they have a wider range of life experiences to draw on. They may have different attitudes to childcare, being more tolerant, patient and better prepared for the demands of being a parent. Having a baby in later life is a positive experience for these women, whether or not the pregnancy was planned (Berryman 1991). Another interesting finding in Berryman's work is that the partners of 'older mothers' are far more likely to be younger than they are. In my view this implies that the expectations and desires of these younger men to father a child are likely to be an important aspect of 'older motherhood'. It also suggests that while some older mothers may be first-time mothers, some may be having a child with a new partner.

The difficulty with Berryman and Windridge's work is that they do not fully analyse the significance and meaning of 'age' but assume chronological age to be a biological fact. So while they conclude that age *per se* does not explain differences between 'older mothers' and younger mothers and that social attitudes play a part, they fail to recognize that the very idea of 'older' and 'younger' mothers is a social construction of 'age'. In a sense they ask the wrong questions; instead of comparing older and younger mothers it is more useful to ask why 'age' is considered important in the first place and why we divide mothers according to age.

Teenage mothers

A discussion of mothers under 20 (the teenage mother) points to why, and how, a woman's age at pregnancy is constructed as significant. Phoenix (1991a, 1991b) shows how teenage pregnancy is frequently linked to suggestions that these young women are seeking welfare benefits and council housing and that their motives for becoming pregnant are 'dubious'. At the same time teenage pregnancy is seen as accidental and irresponsible. In both cases it is the morality of these women which is in question and attitudes towards teenage pregnancy may be seen as an issue of *moral regulation*. In different circumstances competing moral discourses are drawn upon to implicate the 'incompetent' or 'unfit' mother.

Older mothers in Berryman's (1991) analysis make 'good mothers' while very young mothers are 'bad'. Negative attitudes towards teenage mothers when analysed more closely may be understood as expressing a fear that they represent a decline in traditional family values. It is not their age which is the primary issue; rather that these women are more likely to give birth outside marriage. New Right political values emphasize illegitimacy – that is, childbirth outside wedlock – as a major concern (Coufopoulous and Stitt 1994). The **stigmatization** of teenage mothers is therefore linked to the marginalization of unmarried (never married or single) mothers and efforts to control female sexuality (see Chapter 6). In contrast older mothers appear to conform to socially accepted patterns of childbirth and childrearing by not seeing themselves primarily as financial providers and living in heterosexual and traditional types of family settings (see Berryman 1991). What is apparent is that evaluation of 'good mothers' and 'unfit' mothers pivots on these women's relationship to 'the family' and social deprivation.

In the case of teenage mothers the disadvantages which they and their children experience may be attributed to social factors that are only in-directly or unrelated to their age. As Phoenix (1991a) points out poverty is the circumstance for many teenage mothers who are also more likely to be working class, of low educational status, and denied good employment opportunities. Moreover, teenage mothers' view of their own experience of motherhood may be very positive and they do not generally regard themselves as too young to be mothers or as incompetent; neither do they preclude the possibility of marriage at a later date (Phoenix 1991a; 1991b). The prospects for these women are in many respects unchanged by the fact that they have come to motherhood early, since the difficulties they face are common to mothers across age groups.

New reproductive technologies and the 'older woman'

The other area where age and pregnancy has been hotly debated is around the use of new reproductive technologies to assist 'older women' to have a child (see Chapter 7). Once again the positioning of women as 'too old to have a baby' draws on discourses of motherhood which see pregnancy and childbirth as 'natural' processes (Krum 1998). Any suggestion that women might control their own fertility in ways which are 'unnatural' is likely to be contentious, precisely because it challenges the essentialist view that women are their bodies, and because their bodies are subject to social and moral regulation. In order to understand why such strong feelings are expressed about older women giving birth, it is necessary to locate this debate in the context of a broader understanding of how women are constructed as 'old'. Being an 'old' woman by definition is to be regarded as no longer sexually attractive. Since sex and reproduction are commonly tied together (see Chapter 6) the older woman's claim to reproduce is seen as a tenuous and unjustifiable one. In contrast, in a patriarchal and familial society, the (assumed) heterosexuality of (married) women in their twenties automatically qualifies them to become mothers.

Conclusions

Becoming a mother is a significant life event for many, but by no means all women. It is not necessarily central to a woman's life even though it is consistently seen as such and continues to be idealized in popular culture. Attitudes towards becoming a mother are culturally defined and experiences vary. Social position and social identities are interwoven so there is diversity within and between women. For example, women from different ethnic and class backgrounds are likely to have different views of becoming a mother and mothering (Nakano Glenn *et al.* 1994). In Britain, for women from minority ethnic groups, racism constrains the opportunities open to them, shapes their experience of mothering and increases their chances of mothering in poverty. Lesbian and disabled women will also face obstacles to becoming a mother as I shall discuss in the next chapter. Many mothers and their children live in circumstances of poverty and social deprivation.

Women who choose to remain voluntarily child-free are not necessarily selfish or denying their destiny to become mothers. The belief that all women are potential mothers is a cultural myth, an ideological construct, yet it continues to define feminine subjectivity. Mothers are defined in relation to 'others', their identity is simultaneously seen as constituted through their ability to reproduce but also fragmented and dissolved by this very process. Motherhood as a social institution has been constructed around the concept of 'the family'.

Traditionally, marriage and motherhood together created a family. Yet this too is an ideological concept. The stereotypical family is a tool of public policy that has been seen in white culture as historically linked to the rise of the middle classes and increased dependence on wage labour. Theories of childrearing and childcare have changed over time but have frequently positioned the mother at home, looking after the child while the father is at work. These theories supported the idea of 'family' and have shaped family policy for many years.

Today, suggestions that the family is 'in crisis' point to the diversity of experience of women with children. Mothers may be cohabiting, never married, lesbian, divorced or separated, yet social attitudes are slow to change. Fathers still do very little childcare, public provision of childcare is minimal and working mothers continue to be disadvantaged in the workplace. Ideologies of motherhood continue to take hold on the public imagination and women's own view of themselves as mothers continues to be a contradictory one.

There have been changes in feminist thinking about motherhood. In the 1970s motherhood was seen as a site of oppression and many feminists were seen as 'anti-mothers' (Richardson 1993a). Assumptions that (married) women should become mothers, or that 'real women' became 'mothers' were strongly criticized. In the 1980s there was a celebration of motherhood and a view that becoming a mother had the potential to be a positive experience. Moreover there has been, among feminists, an increased recognition of the differences between women and the different circumstances in which women mother. Increasingly, in the 1990s some

women believed that they could 'have it all' and that a career and motherhood could be successfully combined. In practice this represents a continuing daily struggle and brings with it further tensions and contradictions
(Benn 1998). Being a mother is an ambivalent status sometimes idealized
and at other times denigrated and women, including feminists, often feel
ambivalent towards mothering and motherhood (Hollway and Featherstone
1997).

The meaning of motherhood and experiences of mothering have changed
and are changing. The identities of mothers are always unstable. Mothers
experience motherhood in diverse ways and the conditions under which
they mother vary. Being a woman cannot be understood simply in terms
of a capacity to mother or to give birth. Mothering does not come 'naturally' to women and is not the biological destiny of all women. Instead the
identities of mothers and experiences of mothering are historically and
culturally produced. Health care policies and practices that fail to recognize
this are unlikely to be able to meet the health needs of women, mothers
or their children.

The next chapter, in discussing sexual identities, elaborates on this view
of identity as fragmented and discursively produced, rather than being
produced through a stable relationship between ourselves, our bodies and
others. Chapter 7 examines the implications of the new reproductive
technologies for motherhood and whether such developments challenge
conventional beliefs about biological parenthood and women as mothers.

Summary

- This chapter explored the meaning of motherhood and women's experiences of mothering.

- We see here the ways in which mothers and motherhood have been
  'invented'. Discourses of mothering were linked to the knowledge and
  power of the experts who produced theories of mothering and childcare.

- In modern society, the primary role of women has been seen as reproduction. A woman's capacity and potential to bear children has contributed to the view that she is naturally able to care for them. Child-free
  and childless women, and those who cannot care for their child, are
  deemed 'unnatural' or deviant.

- Women's social position has been influenced by attitudes towards the
  family and their role within it. Even the lives of those women who are
  not mothers, or who live outside the traditional, stereotypical family,
  have been shaped by familialism.

- 'The family' has been seen as a tool of public policy which, together
  with ideologies of motherhood, has limited employment opportunities
  for mothers and emphasized their role as childcarers.

- Mother and child health was seen as affected by mothers' exclusion from
  well-paid jobs and the effects of low paid work, poverty and deprivation.

Teenage mothers, black mothers and lone mothers were all seen as particularly vulnerable groups. Their experiences of mothering were seen as structured by negative social attitudes and disadvantage.

- However, the possibility of change is acknowledged. Current concerns about 'a crisis in the family' point to changes in family forms. These changes have also prompted developments in policy. It is too soon to tell whether these developments represent a better future for mothers but there are hopes that women may 'have it all' and may be valued as both mothers and as women.

Discussion points

- In what ways are 'mothers' defined by their relationship to others?
- How have ideas about what constitutes 'the family' shaped attitudes to motherhood?
- Why are 'mothers' regarded as primarily responsible for childcare?
- How difficult is it for women to combine paid employment and domestic work?
- What kinds of explanations are there for the treatment of lone mothers or cohabiting mothers?

Further reading

Ackers, L. and Abbot, P. (1996) *Social Policy for Nurses and the Caring Professions*. Buckingham: Open University Press.

Benn, M. (1998) *Madonna and Child: Towards a New Politics of Motherhood*. London: Jonathan Cape.

Bortolaia Silva, E. (ed.) (1996) *Good Enough Mothering? Feminist Perspectives on Lone Motherhood*. London: Routledge.

Everingham, C. (1994) *Motherhood and Modernity*. Buckingham: Open University Press.

Muncie, J., Wetherell, M., Dallos, R. and Cochrane, A. (eds) (1995) *Understanding the Family*. London: Open University/Sage.

Richardson, D. (1993) *Women, Motherhood and Childrearing*. London: Macmillan.

Utting, D. (1995) *Family and Parenthood: Supporting Families, Preventing Breakdown*. York: Joseph Rowntree Foundation.

VanEvery, J. (1995) *Heterosexual Women Changing the Family: Refusing to be a 'Wife'!* London: Taylor & Francis.

SIX

SEXUAL IDENTITIES

Introduction

In the last chapter I considered what it means to be a mother and mother-hood as a social institution. This chapter explores **sexual identity** and the connections between sex, gender and sexuality. In order to do this I shall examine further the relationship between the biological and the social, between the body and identity. I will discuss how identity is dis-cursively produced and how meanings are inscribed on, or attached to,

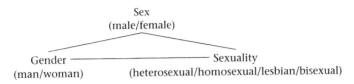

Sex
(male/female)

Gender ———————————— Sexuality
(man/woman)   (heterosexual/homosexual/lesbian/bisexual)

Figure 6.1 Mapping the connections between sex, gender and sexuality

different types of bodies. The categorization of types of bodies and construction of difference are the effects of knowledge and power. Importantly, gender and sexual relations are seen as constructed within specific institutional contexts. The regulation and control of sexuality and gender is tied to scientific approaches to the body and sexual relationships. Medical science in particular has been instrumental in defining what is 'normal' and 'abnormal'.

In this introduction I consider how far existing health care practice addresses issues of sexuality and whether many health professionals take too much for granted. In particular, the extent to which there is a tendency to reinforce heterosexual assumptions, perpetuating certain ideas about what is 'normal' and treating other sexualities as deviant and 'abnormal', or at the very least problematic (Wilton 1997, 1998). The chapter is divided into three sections.

The first section discusses the distinction between sex and gender. This is important because 'patriarchy' rests on a binary divide between male/female, men/women. Such a divide also frequently underpins the organization and delivery of health care. The next section outlines the historical development of theories of sexual difference including pyschoanalytic theory, French feminism, poststructuralism and queer theory. There is a complex debate about the relationship between gender and sexuality that can only be briefly outlined here. This debate is important for understanding why health care practitioners need to separate gender and sexuality. The third section looks at the tying together of sex and reproduction. This underpins the organization of sexuality in modern western society that is characterized by heterosexism. The effect of this is to marginalize those who are not able to reproduce, or who prefer to remain child-free. It also discriminates against those who engage in sexual practices outside a monogamous, heterosexual relationship. The focus of this chapter is therefore the relationship between sex, gender and sexuality and the implications for health care practice (see Figure 6.1).

Health professionals and sexuality

In the first book of its kind, *Sexuality, Nursing and Health*, Webb (1985) broke new ground in proposing that sexuality was important for health care practice. However, Webb's discussion was limited. She focused primarily on gender difference and made only a very brief reference to homosexuality. Lesbian relationships were not discussed at all. Although her intention was to propose that all live according to their own sexual preference, and are unrestricted by gender role, her analysis offered little explanation of how this might become a possibility. Written in the late 1980s, Savage's book, *Nurses, Gender and Sexuality* (1987) describes the reluctance of the nursing profession to engage in discussion about sexuality or to consider the implications for nursing practice. Savage takes the view that 'nursing practice tends unquestioningly to reinforce gender-role' (p. 27) and to link gender and sexuality even though 'gender identity does not necessarily determine sexual practice' (p. 20). She argues that nurses should challenge gender stereotypes and dominant definitions of what it means to be a man or a woman, rather than perpetuate gender divisions and hierarchies (p. 139).

Nearly ten years later, Christine Webb (1994) suggests that things have moved on, that nurses have begun to talk about sexuality. However several of the papers in her volume appear to see sexuality primarily within a medical framework or as a nursing problem (Jones and Webb 1994; Meerabeau 1994). The contributors also report a low level of awareness of sexual issues among health care practitioners, unwillingness to discuss sex with client groups (Faugier 1994), **homophobia**, discrimination and gender stereotyping (Ferguson 1994; Turton 1994). In particular there are reports of a continuing reluctance of nursing professionals to meet the health care needs of lesbian women in the UK (Brogan 1997) and the USA (Waterhouse 1996; Walpin 1997). At the same time there is a growing expectation that nurses have an important role in promoting sexual health (Irwin 1997).

Writing for midwives, Symonds and Hunt (1996) discuss social aspects of motherhood and say 'the interlinking of sexual identity, sexual activity and motherhood is a very complex tangle to unpick' (p. 118). They say lesbian sexuality is frequently presented in opposition to motherhood: 'If motherhood is the desire of all "natural" and "real" women, how does one explain the lesbian mother? Either lesbianism is a part of being a "natural" woman or motherhood is not, this is the inescapable and logical dilemma posed by a rigid definition of femininity and motherhood' (p. 119).

This raises many questions about the connections between gender, sexuality and motherhood. Walton (1994), a midwife, provides a more detailed discussion of sexuality and motherhood for midwives, and draws on sociological work. She provides a useful account of the construction of sexuality and refers to the prejudices and discrimination that lesbian women frequently experience in maternity services. This is seen in the context of a society where legal, medical and other social institutions are characterized as homophobic. Midwives are described as reluctant to discuss sexuality or to consider the connections between sexuality and motherhood. However, while recognizing that sexuality is socially constructed, contradictorily Walton takes for granted the biological basis of sexuality and ties together sex, gender and sexuality. Much of her discussion of pregnancy and childbirth assumes that the woman is heterosexual.

The issues are complex and my aim here is to point to the sociological literature that relates to key debates in this area and to try to sketch out what these are. I hope this will provide some means of advancing discussion among midwives and nurses about the meaning of sexual identity and its implication for health care, especially in relation to pregnancy and childbirth. Symonds and Hunt (1996), Walton (1994) and Savage (1987) all suggest that midwives and nurses tend to 'fall into the trap of assuming that all women are heterosexual, married and happy to be mothers' (Symonds and Hunt 1996: 119). So, my starting point is that there is a need to rethink the links between motherhood and sexuality and between fatherhood and sexuality. This also means rethinking the links between sex and reproduction so as to uncouple them and see sexual pleasure as separate from reproduction (Hawkes 1996). By doing so it becomes easier to identify why heterosexist ideologies permeate health care and to consider ways in which health care professionals, including nurses, midwives and doctors, might improve their practice.

Sex and gender

In contemporary western society there is a widely held view that biological differences are uncontested and self-evident (see Haraway 1991 for an important discussion of this point). Such an ideology pervades much of the media representations of sex and sexuality in film, popular journals and elsewhere. Men and women are frequently represented in ways that reinforce heterosexist notions of *femininity* and *masculinity*. Put simply, the ideal feminine woman is seen as weak, passive and beautiful while the masculine man is represented as strong and active with a muscular body. Such images represent a dichotomous world view where sex differences between male and female are used to frame gender and the sexual identities of men and women. A binary divide between men and women is set up which in turn supports heterosexual relations and patriarchal society. The concept of patriarchy has been much debated in feminist theory (see Chapter 4) and I use the term here within the framework of a binary split between men and women as a particular historical formation. However the proposal by Hooper (1997) (discussed below) to talk of 'a masculinist culture' does seem to be more useful in drawing out the differences between men and the ways in which discourses, institutions and bodies intersect.

The debates about sex and gender are around the relationship between nature (the biological) and culture (the social). Within feminist theory there has been a continuing debate about the significance and meaning of biological 'sex' differences. While some argued for a distinction between biological sex and gender as a social construct, others reduced gender to sex. So for the former, what it means to be woman or man was seen as the result of socialization and cultural processes not the result of 'nature'. For the latter, there were important 'natural' differences between the sexes that needed to be recognized and valued. In the 1970s the distinction between sex and gender was widely accepted.

Identity politics

For many feminists the political effectiveness of a collective gender identity has been strategically important (Stanley and Wise 1993; Assiter 1996). Gender theory, especially in the 1970s and 1980s, which highlighted the social construction of gender and (sexual) difference was important for underpinning feminist struggles for equality and liberation. However, more recently in feminist theory the need to recognize differences between women has highlighted the heterosexist assumptions that were central to earlier struggles. Arguably, regarding women as an **homogenous** group, disadvantaged in contemporary society, failed to account for other forms of discrimination linked, for example, to ethnicity, sexuality, class and disability. The merits of identity politics, a political struggle based on a shared and collective identity, increasingly came under scrutiny (Spelman 1988; see also Chapter 3). Increasingly feminists argued against such a sex/gender distinction saying that this perpetuated a dualistic and hetero-sexist view of social life (Wilkinson and Kitzinger 1993a; 1993b; Assiter 1996; Richardson 1996a). Instead others (for example Butler 1993) argued that 'sex' is not simply, in reductionist or essentialist terms, a matter of biological difference but itself may be seen as *constructed*.

The extent to which it is useful to talk of women sharing a collective identity is frequently characterized as a polarized debate between uni-versal essentialism and social constructionism. There are however a range of positions on this issue (see for example, Jackson *et al.* 1993; Jackson and Scott 1996) and it has been suggested that essentialism and construc-tionism are not polar opposites at all (Fuss 1989).

However, put simply:

- An *essentialist* view of sexuality is that sexuality, though shaped by social processes, derives from 'natural' biological bodily processes. According to this view there is a fixed biological essence of (sexual) being. Identity is naturalized and linked to bodily form. The materiality (physicality) of the body is emphasized.
- A *social constructionist* view of sexuality argues that historical and cul-tural processes construct or create the meaning of sexuality. This chal-lenges the notion that biology underpins sexuality and instead attaches greater importance to social processes. In Foucauldian terms 'identity' is seen as an unstable product of discourses (knowledge and power) that in turn give meaning to bodies. The relationship between bodies and identity is seen as dynamic and changing.

So what is gender?

The relationship between the *symbolic* and the *material* (physical) body is a complex one and much debated (see also Chapter 8). Gatens (1996) asks 'What is gender?' And what is the distinction between sex and gender? 'Sex is typically understood as a biological given and gender as a social construction which overlays this biology' (1996: 31). Yet frequently the term gender displaces sex. In Gatens' discussion of feminist theory, the emphasis on gender in the feminist politics of the 1970s and 1980s in effect portrayed the body as a neutral entity. By emphasizing socialization processes in the formation of gender identities the connection between sex and gender came to be seen as arbitrary and the differences between the male and female body ignored. For Gatens, such a view of the body is **rationalist**, separating consciousness (mind) from the body in a way which fails to take into account the lived experiences of female bodies as distinct from male bodies. An emphasis on socialization also posits the mind as a *tabula rasa* (Gatens 1996: 16).

The differences between male and female bodies are, in the view of Gatens (1996), historical fact. This she says does *not* imply a form of essentialism, in that the relationship between sex and gender is not fixed, but neither is it arbitrary. It is linked historically, according to how social value and meaning attaches to different types of bodies. Gatens argues therefore that the sex/gender distinction made in those earlier accounts needs reconsidering: 'Rather I would suggest that "masculinity" and "femininity" correspond at the level of the imaginary body to "male" and "female" at the level of biology. It bears repeating that this statement does not imply a fixed essence to "masculine" and "feminine" but rather a historical specificity' (Gatens 1996: 16). For Gatens, sexual politics cannot therefore be reconstructed in terms of gender differences but sexual difference remains important because it is women's *bodies* that are engaged in struggle and political conflict.

Gatens argues that in **phallocentric culture** – that is, at the level of the symbolic or the imaginary – the construction of sexual and gender difference into a 'normative dualism of two bodies, two sexes and two genders' ('masculine' or 'feminine') denies the possibility of multiple body types and diverse identifications:

> The **polymorphous** body need not be divided strictly into two kinds: male and female. Indeed, it is this strict division that is the insignia of patriarchy . . . The gendered body images of male and female – that which allows them to 'live' as sexed men and women – are body doubles. To insist on this difference, in *all* contexts as *the* difference, is to confess to one's fascination with the double.
>
> (Gatens 1996: 43, original emphasis)

Though 'doubling' is a useful idea in psychoanalytic theory to explain the process of identity formation, Gatens says that the repeated opposition and complementarity of the 'masculine' and 'feminine' is a feature of phallocentric culture. So how can we move beyond this dualism and heterosexist ideology?

Masculinities

Connell (1995) is also critical of this dualism in his discussion of men's bodies and bodily practices. Drawing on the work of Connell (1987) Hooper (1997: 19) offers a useful approach to gender theory. She explains that: 'gender is neither a thing nor a property of individual character. It is a property of collectivities, institutions and historical processes. It is also a linking concept whereby biological difference is engaged with and social practices are organised'. So, following Connell, she argues for a process of 'engendering' which creates the possibility of 'multiple interpretations of gender'. Rather than seeing gender identity in terms of a simple division between men and women, the masculine and the feminine, what it means to be a man or woman is variable and diverse. Gender identity cannot be reduced to biological sex difference but instead sexed bodies, male and female, are historically and socially produced. By seeing identities as fluid, dynamic and changing, 'masculinity' (and femininity) may be seen to take many forms and to be integrated with other identities.

What Hooper's (1997) analysis does is to explore the construction of gender identity along three dimensions of the body, institutions and discourses. She discusses how, within what she calls a 'masculinist culture', certain types of bodies, institutional forms and discourses interact, which both constitutes (produces) subjects and positions them. In western culture white, heterosexual, middle-class men embody 'hegemonic masculinity' and are positioned in a hierarchy above other men and above women. This enables these men to enjoy the privileges attached to this form of masculinity that are less accessible to other men (or women). Such an approach therefore helps to explain similarities and differences between men and between men and women, not simply in terms of sexual difference but in terms of the extent to which they are able to identify with dominant forms of masculinity.

In Hooper's terms 'masculinism' best describes the gender order in which masculinity is privileged rather than men. Not all men are equal and in this masculinist culture where heterosexism, racism and other axes of oppression operate, 'hegemonic masculinity' links power and status to heterosexuality and penetrative sex, but also class and ethnicity. Hooper (1997) suggests that class, gender and sexuality intersect and that identities are always *racialized* (see also Spelman 1988; Collins 1993; Bahvnani 1997). Heterosexuality is defined in opposition to homosexuality and gay men are subordinate to straight men. Through similar processes black men are marginalized by 'hegemonic masculinity'. For these men especially, and for other groups who are oppressed and marginalized, identity is not experienced as unitary but is more likely to be fragmented, contradictory and confusing (Hooper 1997: 20). These power relations are not static but dynamic, constantly subject to negotiation and change, which contributes to this uncertainty and instability. Identities are always contingent and in a state of flux – what Ferguson (1993) refers to as 'mobile subjectivities'. It is in this Foucauldian sense that power is productive, producing and constituting subject positions but then appearing to fix and naturalize them.

If we accept then that sex, gender and sexuality are not reducible to (or in a fixed relation to) each other, it follows that the experiences of men and women in relation to reproduction are not uniform. For example, we cannot make assumptions that homosexual men have chosen not to become fathers, any more than we can see a lesbian sexual identity as contradictory to being a mother (see Chapters 5 and 7).

Gender and sexuality

Historical organization of sexuality

Ideas about sexual difference have changed over time and views of sexual difference are historical. Christian values have been influential but also, as part of the secularization of society (Turner 1995), science has played an increasingly important role in regulating sexual (social) behaviour. The **scientific paradigm** defined sexual matters as biological ones. Biology was the scientific study of the human organism and sexuality was seen in biological terms (Haraway 1991; Hawkes 1996; Segal 1997). Sexual difference was understood as difference between the male and female body. Despite evidence to the contrary that suggested many similarities between male and female bodies, differences, especially in external genitalia, were highlighted. The reasons for such differences being emphasized may be seen as primarily connected with social, political and economic changes in the modern world. Turner (1992, 1995), Foucault (1979, 1985, 1990), Weeks (1981, 1985, 1991) and Hawkes (1996) suggest that the organization of sexuality and the regulation of sexual behaviour must be understood in the context of the cultural shifts of the time.

In Europe, during Victorian times, patriarchal values produced a view of women's sexuality as particularly problematic. Concerns about regulating populations were translated into controls over women's sexual behaviour (Turner 1995). Women were seen as 'guardians of the race' and 'vampires upon the nation's health', both asexual and yet sexually dangerous (Segal 1997: 190). Such views shaped the kinds of medical treatments and health care made available to women whose frequent 'hysterical' behaviour was attributed to dysfunction of the female reproductive organs and necessitated hysterectomy as a corrective (Turner 1995). At the same time these ideas supported a gender hierarchy based on dichotomous thinking which created a binary divide between male/female, masculine/feminine, active/passive. This binary opposition has supported heterosexual ideology since that time (Weeks 1985) and also, as I shall discuss below, linked together sex, marriage and reproduction (see also Chapter 5).

The biomedical tradition

The biomedical tradition pathologized female sexuality outside marriage and this pathologization (mis)informed ideas about health and disease. **Sexology** – the science of sex – underpinned this tradition by attempting to identify ' "natural" sexuality, directed towards procreative ends, from its "unnatural" or "perverse" forms – homosexuality, sadism, rape and lust murder' (Segal 1997: 191). However, according to Matus (1995) studies of Victorian 'sexual science' have overemphasized 'the rigid categorisation of men and women as fundamentally different'. She argues instead that 'the biomedical responses to the question of sexual difference were never unanimous or univocal' (1995: 5). In her view these debates, in Victorian times, about what was 'natural' indicated the instability of nature and the potential effects of social interference. So, for example, the idea that the education of women would have a detrimental effect on their reproductive capacity was illustrative of the ways in which social factors were thought to influence biological functioning. It follows therefore that questions of sexual difference were extremely vexed and that bodies may be seen as much more unstable than the rigid categorizations of male and female suggested (Matus 1995).

Since that time, there have been disputes about whether later attempts by sexologists to acknowledge the possibility of female sexual pleasure, in addition to male sexual pleasure, advanced a more positive view of women or simply reinforced gender divisions (Segal 1994, 1997; Smart 1997). In so far as it went beyond a view of sexuality as essentially linked to reproduction and focused on sexual pleasure, sexology was liberatory (Hawkes 1996; Segal 1997). However, sexualized racist metaphors also gained prominence at that time creating negative racist stereotypes of black men (Hall 1997b) and black women (Gilman 1985; Collins 1993). These ideas continue to have currency in contemporary society though new challenges to them have arisen.

At the theoretical level, challenges to this biological reductionism have come from psychoanalysis, feminism, social construction and queer theory. While there is dispute about the implications of psychoanalysis, it has been seen as going beyond the physiological model of gender and sexuality 'to explore the symbolic and psychic meanings' (Segal 1997: 196). (But see also Mitchell 1974; Millett 1977; Chodorow 1978; Hawkes 1996.) Feminism sought to undermine gender hierarchies, while social construction and queer theory explore more fully ideas about plural sexualities and the formation of sexual identities as socially contingent; as products of regulatory social processes which may be resisted.

Freud to Foucault

The influence of Freud (1961, 1986) on our thinking about sex is well known (Payne and Walker 1996). Freud's theories (see Box 6.1) could be

---

Box 6.1   Freud – a key thinker

According to Freud, sexual drives could take many forms and be directed towards many objects. This he related to early childhood experiences of pleasure and pain. The repression of these drives as a result of disturbances, or obstacles encountered, formed the unconscious. Sexuality did not relate to anatomy directly since any area of the body could produce sexual pleasure. In theorizing sexual difference Freud 'explained' femininity and masculinity in terms of the different relationship of the boy and girl child to the mother and father – the Oedipal dramas.

Freud does seem to be assuming some sort of fixed polarity in sexual difference. Homosexuality is thus fundamentally (although again contradictions and inconsistencies abound) a mixed-up form of heterosexuality (Segal 1997: 199). Arguably, despite relocating sexuality in the mind, Freud continued to reduce sexual difference to biology.

Key texts for Freud include:
The Standard Edition of the Complete Psychological Works of Sigmund Freud (1961) and *On Sexuality: Three Essays on the Theory of Sexuality and Other Works* (1986).

seen as a shift away from thinking about sex in biological terms (the biological drives and instincts of the sexologists): 'The psychoanalytic account of sexuality was elaborated with concepts describing a different site of sexual reality: "psychic" or internal mental life, and the centrality of the unconscious, or repressed memories within it' (Segal 1997: 196). However, feminist criticisms of Freud's work suggest that he reproduced and strengthened heterosexist thinking and that his views of female sexuality were very negative, based on the idea of a lack (of a penis) (see Mitchell 1974; Millett 1977; Chodorow 1978; Grosz 1995).

Psychoanalytic thought has continued to shape debate especially in France. Lacan, a French psychoanalyst, 'theorized subjectivity as constructed in and through *language*, within a symbolic order in which "the phallus is the privileged signifier"' (Segal 1997: 200, my emphasis). So, rather than a biological reductionist position being adopted by Lacan, his work is seen as emphasizing the **symbolic**, linguistic and discursive production of subjectivity. However, whether feminists may usefully take up these ideas is hotly debated (Richardson 1997).

The influential theorist, Foucault (1979, 1985, 1990), offers a view of sexuality which contrasts with both psychoanalytic and biomedical accounts. As already indicated in Chapter 2 Foucault's concern was to propose an historical, cultural analysis of knowledge and power. His view of sexuality, much discussed since, was to see the 'problem' of sexuality as linked to the problem of government and regulation. The very idea that sexuality is a problem, in Foucauldian terms, may be seen as socially constructed. The disciplining, or regulating, of sexual behaviour and morality itself are constituted in this way as problems of social control. Heterosexist ideology therefore has the political and moral effect of promoting sex between men and women, of patterning sexual behaviour according to **social norms** (Smart 1997; Wilkinson and Kitzinger 1993a, 1993b; Richardson 1996a, 1996b). At the same time, homosexual and lesbian sexualities are constituted as marginal, deviant and 'immoral'.

Foucault's project (at least, one of them) was to show how discourses of modernity shaped and produced an historically specific cultural landscape. He says the body is inscribed with social meanings that construct desires, pleasures and sexualities. According to such a view, heterosexual and homosexual desires are constructed from a multiplicity of discourses. Sexual identities, rather than being tied to biology or some inner essence, are discursively produced. Professional discourses including medicine, nursing and midwifery are implicated in Foucault's analysis because it is these discourses which seek to label, classify and identify pathologies and abnormalities, marking difference and defining what is normal.

French feminism and poststructuralism

So, we need to understand that identity, rather than being tied to biological givens, may be seen as unstable, fluid and discursively produced. The symbolic world, or language used to talk about who (or what) we are, is socially produced and connects the personal and public spheres. So although gender identities *appear* naturalized and directly tied to biology, this is the effect of discourses of modernity, the humanist project to locate the subject of history. Foucault proposed a view of identity formation that was *anti-essentialist* because it denied the pre-existence of an essence of being or a biological given. Instead the contingent and historical production of identities such as woman/man, straight/gay were seen as produced by discourse.

The way in which meaning is inscribed on bodies and identity is constructed is through *representational practices*. These include the spoken word and a variety of media such as books, photographs, film and magazines (see Chapter 8). Feminists have for some time drawn attention to how women are represented and have taken issue with the work of Freud, Lacan and Foucault. The extent to which their theories are useful in advancing feminist projects has been a matter of controversy (Assiter 1996; Sawicki 1991; McNay 1992). French feminists in particular have been engaged with exploring the potentialities of re-conceptualizing the female subject and 'speaking as a woman' – that is, finding alternative ways of representing or signifying 'woman'. The work of Luce Irigaray (1985a, 1985b) has been important in this debate (see Box 6.2).

Box 6.2 Irigaray – a key thinker

Luce Irigaray is a French feminist philosopher. She draws on psychoanalytic ideas. In her writing, Irigaray attempts to explore **sexual politics** at the level of the symbolic. For her, the subjugation of women is achieved by silencing women. Women are excluded from political life because they have no voice. The language of politics offers no space for women because, in language, women are consistently reduced to their sex; reduced to biology. The female subject therefore is constituted in specific ways that effectively exclude her from political life. The very concept of an autonomous subject with bodily integrity is, according to this view, masculinist and exclusionary. In contrast, women's bodies are represented as lacking both autonomy and integrity. In phallocentric culture, women lack the phallus that represents power, integrity and subjecthood.

Irigaray's most famous works include:
Speculum of the Other Woman (1985a) and *This Sex which is not One* (1985b).

A useful introduction to her ideas is Whitford, M. (1991) *Luce Irigaray: Philosopher in the Feminine*. London: Routledge. See also Fuss, D. (1989) *Essentially Speaking: Feminism, Nature and Difference*. London: Routledge.

However, other feminists are critical of Irigaray's project suggesting that a sexual politics which attempts to speak *through* women's bodies essentializes women, once more reducing them to biology and implying a fixed essence to the feminine subject (Butler 1990). This criticism is contentious

(Fuss 1989; Whitford, 1991) and may miss the point. If language excludes women, representing and constituting them in specific ways, the possibility of an alternative language raises the possibility of multiple voices, new ways of speaking and wider participation in political life. Such a possibility may reconfirm sexual difference but need not necessarily regard such differences as fixed or immutable.

Lesbian feminism and queer theory

In *Bodies that Matter: On the Discursive Limits of Sex* Butler (1993) argues that nature (sex) is not simply acted upon by culture, and also against the idea that radical constructionism loses sight of the **materiality** of the body. To say that the body is discursively produced is not necessarily to imply that the body has no materiality. Rather, according to Butler, the materialization of 'sex' is discursively constituted. Materialization is produced, not fixed, but constantly reiterated. Repetition of these processes to constitute sex also provides the possibility of variation and change, so although 'sex' appears natural, a given, it is produced historically, over time. The connections between sex, gender and sexuality may therefore be loosened; one cannot simply be read off from another. 'Sex' is not, in Butler's view, pre-discursive or outside discourse but the very notion of a 'natural sex' or 'sexed nature' is culturally produced. Matus (1995) criticizes Butler for conflating sex and gender but this seems to be a misreading of Butler's intention. Butler wants to unsettle the distinction between sex (biology) and gender (culture) but she does not say that sex and gender are the same.

The implications of Butler's work and this untying of sex and gender allows for diverse sexual identities. For as long as sexual difference is thought of in terms of a binary divide between 'male' and 'female' it supports gender identities of 'man' and 'woman'. Once these divisions are seen as culturally produced, as historical and tied to the discourses of modernity and patriarchy, the alternatives come into view. 'Queer theory', by taking up the ideas of Foucault, historicizes lesbian and gay identities (Fuss 1989; Stacey 1997). A cultural or sociological perspective points to the normative, homophobic assumptions and discourses of dominant social groups who position homosexual and lesbian identities as on the margins and as deviant. Such discourses fail to recognize the polymorphous body or diverse forms of desires and pleasures. Within heterosexist discourse the desire of one woman for another cannot be understood, or explained, for heterosexuality presupposes that the female subject is constituted in opposition to, and complementary to, the male. Heterosexual 'sex' (heterosex) by definition is sex between a man and a woman (Rich 1980; Wilkinson and Kitzinger 1993a, 1993b; Richardson 1996a, 1996b). Sex between women, or between men, disrupts this binary division and is marked as transgressive and contradictory. For lesbian feminists, as for many other feminists but in different ways, the body is a site for struggle and resistance. Lesbian feminists and queer theorists challenge ideas about what is 'normal' sexuality. But the relationship between their ideas is complex and there are differences of view about political strategy and what it means to be a lesbian (or gay) (Fuss 1989; Wilton 1995; Stacey 1997).

This discussion of sexual difference has shown that the connections between bodies, discourses and institutions are complex. There are different types of bodies but the emphasis on differences between male and female bodies is historical and socially constructed. In recognizing the effects of social processes – how, for example, biological and medical scientific discourses and institutions of government construct typologies of male/female, normal/abnormal sexual behaviour – we need not deny the materiality of bodies. It is bodies which have desires, perform sexual acts and give birth but in so doing they **embody** social practices. Sexual identities and gender identities relate to bodily difference but not in a fixed or predetermining way. Instead, 'identities' are constantly being produced; they are socially contingent.

Sex and reproduction

In the introduction to this chapter I suggested that contemporary health care practice continues to reinforce heterosexist ideologies. Calls for a return to family values and to discourage sex outside marriage even today reinforce heterosexist and conservative ideologies based on biological reductionism (see Chapter 5). What continues is the tendency for many health care practitioners and others to link together sex and reproduction (Wilton 1997). This, according to Hawkes (1996) is a feature of 'modernist sexuality'.

Civilization and rationalization

By adopting an historical and sociological perspective of sex and sexuality, Hawkes (1996) describes how attitudes have changed and developed, but also what she calls the 'threads of continuity'. Her analysis draws on the work of Elias, Freud and Weber in order to explain how sex and reproduction came to be linked. She explains that Elias' notion of the **civilizing process** describes how restraint and the containment of feelings and desires became important in modern life.

Sexual activity, like other forms of social behaviour such as eating, was publicly acknowledged and recognized in the pre-modern era. Increasingly however there was an enlargement of the 'private' spheres of life, increased feelings of shame and embarrassment associated with sexual activity, and the bedroom was no longer a public space. Freud also saw a tension between 'civilization' and sexuality which led to the repression of what came to be regarded as animalistic behaviour, incestuous desire and childhood sexuality (Hawkes 1996). The social theorist, Weber, explained this with reference to the process of rationalization. Modern society comprised a new social order that was produced and sustained by the rationalizing of social life. This meant that the 'irrational' desires and pleasures of sexual behaviour increasingly became routinized and constrained. Sexual pleasure became routinized through the institution of heterosexual marriage (see Chapter 5).

So, in Hawkes' account, from the eighteenth century heterosexual desire became the primary legitimate means of sexual pleasure in the form of penetrative, conjugal, procreative sex. Although 'Enlightenment sexuality' celebrated male sexual pleasure this celebration was within strictly defined limits and 'healthy sex' was *reproductive sex* between a man and a woman. There remained, as I have already outlined in Chapter 5, a continued ambivalence about women's sexuality and the sexuality of the young and the lower classes.

Moral regulation

The new morality associated with industrial capitalism and the rise of the bourgeois society created a context for even tighter moral regulation and legal control over sexual behaviour. Sexuality was both class-based and gender-based, and the claims of women and the working classes for political rights represented a threat to male power and masculinity (Hawkes 1996). Male power (patriarchy), as already indicated, was directly tied to concepts of **hegemonic masculinity** and heterosexuality. Homosexuality and other forms of non-procreative sex became increasingly marginalized and regarded as morally reprehensible and illegitimate:

> The increasing focus on sexual practices led to the creation of a sexual centre of heterosexuality with a hinterland of practitioners of non-procreative sex. These separate sexual spheres were populated by 'figures' who represented sexual ideals to be strived for: the monogamous heterosexual conjugal couple, the innocent child, the sexually dependent and pure woman.
>
> (Hawkes 1996: 48)

It follows from this analysis that the rise of pro-natalist ideologies and the medicalization of pregnancy and childbirth outlined in Chapter 2 were closely related to prevailing attitudes towards sex and sexuality.

Controlling women

Women were increasingly defined as sexual objects, the objects of male desire, and were considered primarily destined to reproduce. Their sexuality and sexual activity was considered only in relation to men and their *raison d'être* was reproduction and mothering. It is in this context that controversies about the use of contraception, abortion and, more recently, new reproductive technologies (see Chapter 7) must be understood. The extent to which reproduction and mothering is regarded as the essence of 'woman' shapes the views of diverse groups in relation to these debates. Hawkes (1996) outlines the uneasy alliances between medical professionals, feminists, social commentators and Fabian socialists towards the extended use of birth control. For some, contraception could release women from the suffering and burden associated with numerous pregnancies, and liberate their sexuality. While for others, the promise of sexual pleasure without the possibility of pregnancy signalled a lapse in standards of moral and social behaviour and even the potential exploitation of women as sexual slaves. Although state planning of reproduction and policies for population control were increasingly regarded as necessary, the direction and implications of practices of birth control were contentious. Hence the initial restriction of contraception for married women reflected the view that only conjugal sexual activity was legitimate.

Similar controversies surround the intervention of the state today in formulating public policy in sexual and reproductive matters. Controversies have arisen around compulsory sterilization of women deemed mentally or socially unfit to be mothers (Doyal 1995), court orders for Ceasarean section, the rights of fathers to prevent abortion of an unborn foetus and the limited availability of infertility treatment for some women (Wilton 1997). The idea that women might control their own fertility and reproductive lives has been tied to ideas about sexual promiscuity and licence. Women taking control over their lives represented a threat to the social order that kept women in their place – at home looking after children. Pregnancy and childbirth even today are often regarded as a woman's biological destiny. The social, political, economic and historical conditions that link together sex, gender and sexuality position women in a hierarchy where the heterosexual, married mother is regarded as fulfilling her biological destiny. Other women, including teenage women, women with disabilities and lesbian women are seen as potentially dangerous and marginal, and are frequently discouraged, or prevented, from reproducing (Wilton 1997).

Teenage sex

Teenage sex is consistently defined as problematic. A recent conversation with a colleague reminded me of how my own experience of teenage pregnancy in the 1970s was illustrative of that time. The very idea that teenage girls might be engaged in sexual activity was controversial and access to 'family planning clinics' or contraception via the GP was difficult and a matter for concealment. As a pregnant teenager I was considered a 'high risk' and often contact with health professionals included unwelcome and unwanted advice on how to behave. Twenty-five years on, teenage sexuality continues to be seen as 'a problem' and a brief literature search reveals a number of writers addressing this (Lees 1993; Webb 1994; Jannke 1996; Safe Motherhood 1996; Tilsey 1997).

Evidently the legal and social concept of 'the child' which developed in modern society and became divorced from sexuality created a particular difficulty with respect to acknowledging the emotional and physical capacity of teenagers for sexual activity. Teen pregnancy is still usually regarded as unplanned and uncontrolled, if not unwanted.

For many women teenage sex marks the early recognition (perhaps only in retrospect) of the expectation that their fertility is subject to control. While contraception is one means of control, another is abortion. Paradoxically perhaps, the teenage girl may subsequently be seen as acting

---

Box 6.3   Teenage pregnancy in the UK

- The UK is reported as having the highest rate of teen pregnancy in the developed world (Nolan 1998).
- Figures for 1990 show that Britain has the highest birth rate in western Europe but figures from the USA are even higher. The teenage conception rate in Britain is also the highest in western Europe and has risen since 1980 unlike elsewhere (Health Education Authority 1994).
- In 1997 the UK government set up four task groups to develop an action plan to tackle 'the problem of teenage pregnancy' (Nolan 1998).
- 1992 figures for abortion in the UK show a decline overall since the early 1980s. The majority of abortions are carried out for women aged between 20–30 years old. However the number of teenagers having abortions has increased and this is attributed to poor access to family planning services (Health Education Authority 1994).

---

responsibly in seeking an abortion, when this is a less favoured option for married women. Certainly in the early 1970s giving birth outside wedlock was as problematic as having an abortion, though the legalization of abortion in limited circumstances, and other social changes, may be seen as influencing contemporary attitudes to teenage pregnancy and sexuality (see Box 6.3).

Controlling fertility and abortion

In her book *Abortion and Woman's Choice* Petchesky (1986) outlines the social and economic changes which help to explain the numbers of predominantly teenage women seeking abortion in the USA. She explains that the changing attitudes of women towards marriage relates to the growing numbers of teenage women seeking abortions since the 1970s and the rising number of births outside wedlock. However, such trends among teenage women, in her view, are linked to broader social changes not an 'epidemic of adolescent pregnancy' (Petchesky 1986: 211). For her, the political and economic gains for many women (in the USA) since that time enabled them to 'choose' abortion, to marry later and gain financial independence through participation in employment. Legalized abortion and contraception could be seen as enabling for women, allowing them to control their own fertility and explore their sexuality. Although Petchesky sees the level of advantages for different groups of women as variable, especially black women, increasingly there was a democratization of sexuality among women in the USA. Both black and white young women became identified as sexually active where previously 'promiscuity' was associated mainly with marginalized groups rather than white, middle-class women.

Box 6.4 Abortion law in Britain since 1990

The conditions which have to be met for a legal abortion to be performed under the terms of the Act:

A there is a threat to the life of the pregnant woman, greater than if the pregnancy were terminated; or

B the termination is necessary to prevent grave permanent injury to the physical or mental health of the pregnant woman; or

C the pregnancy has not exceeded its twenty-fourth week and that the continuance of the pregnancy would involve risk, greater than if the pregnancy were terminated, or injury to the physical or mental health of the pregnant woman; or

D the pregnancy has not exceeded its twenty-fourth week and that the continuance of the pregnancy would involve risk, greater than if the pregnancy were terminated, of injury to the physical or mental health of any existing child(ren) of the family of the pregnant woman; or

E there is a substantial risk that if the child were born it would suffer from such physical and mental abnormalities as to be seriously handicapped.

There are no time limits for clauses A, B and E.

Source: Brien and Fairbairn (1996: 40).

In Britain 'abortion is the most frequently performed operation inside and outside the NHS' (Brien and Fairbairn 1996: 38). In 1995, 66 per cent of voters in a MORI poll supported 'abortion on request' (Brien and Fairbairn 1996). Yet abortion continues to be a contentious issue. Campaigns to reduce the time limit within which abortions may be legally performed resulted in amendments to the 1967 Abortion Act in 1990 (see also Box 6.4 and Chapter 7): 'The 1967 Abortion Act, amended by the 1990 Human Fertilisation & Embryology Act, lays down the principal conditions which allow a registered medical practitioner to perform an abortion once two independent doctors have agreed' (Brien and Fairbairn 1996: 40).

'Abortions have to be carried out in an NHS hospital or approved place' (Brien and Fairbairn 1996: 41). In Northern Ireland abortions are illegal, except to save the life of the mother or where the pregnancy would involve 'serious injury to her physical or mental health' (Brien and Fairbairn 1996: 41). Irish women (those from both Northern Ireland and the Irish Republic) seeking abortions travel to England for a private abortion – an estimated 4154 women did so in 1991. In 1994, 1678 women from Northern Ireland travelled to England for an abortion. These figures do not include others who obtained access to an NHS abortion (Brien and Fairbairn 1996: 41). The majority (110,384 or 66 per cent) of all women seeking abortion in the UK are single (see Table 6.1). The availability of NHS

Table 6.1 Marital status of those women (resident and non-resident) seeking abortion in England and Wales in 1994

Marital status	Number of women
Single	110,384
Married	36,135
Widowed	499
Divorced	7,615
Separated	6,424
Not stated	5,819
Total	166,876

Source: OPCS, Monitors AB 95/8 in Brien and Fairbairn (1996).

abortion services and access to reliable information varies and may be affected by where a woman lives. Private charities also provide abortion services for a variable fee.

Although there are cultural differences between Britain and the USA, and contrasting institutional forms of health care which Petchesky (1986) acknowledges, she argues that her analysis does offer some potential insights into the British experience. In Britain, as in the USA, there is a view that a sexual revolution occurred in the 1970s and feminists have been important in campaigning for reproductive freedom. Moreover she argues that abortion is at the centre of a struggle around the meanings of the family, the state, motherhood and young women's sexuality. Such a struggle has occurred in the British context and in the absence of careful comparative work between the USA and Britain at the time she was writing, her insights are useful.

The idea that the availability of contraception and abortion resulted in a liberalization of teenage sexual behaviour is, according to Petchesky, problematic. She suggests a more complex picture. She argues that the actions, attitudes and beliefs of teenage girls reproduce heterosexist culture. Teenage girls have engaged in heterosexual activity as part of the process of defining their sexual identities. The pressures to conform to heterosexist cultural norms, to acquire a feminine sexual identity, while at the same time resist sexual activity and prevent pregnancy, are contradictory for young women. Moreover, in Petchesky's view, sexual activity in adolescence provides a source of power in processes of individuation and separation of young women from their families. The availability of abortion and contraception contributed to the rise of a new consciousness about women's sexuality. This impacted on the previously accepted connections between sex and marriage but reinforced an heterosexual identity for women (Petchesky 1986). Sex without reproduction has always been a possibility, but the evidence on abortion and contraceptive use made heterosexual activity (specifically intercourse) more visible (Petchesky 1986).

Fertility control has also been directed at specific groups of women rather than universally encouraged: 'most national governments have more complex agendas, often involving attempts to maintain or restructure existing social divisions' (Doyal 1995: 98). Concerns about population size have always been linked, more or less explicitly, to the composition of the population. Historically, during the early part of the twentieth century in the UK and across Europe, the **eugenics** movement enjoyed some support among social reformers and concerns about the fertility of the working classes were not the same as concerns about middle-class women (Spallone 1992). In Chapter 7 I discuss whether attitudes and policies surrounding the use of new reproductive technologies and the development of the 'new genetics' today may be framed (perhaps unintentionally) in similar ways. These developments may be seen as shaping attitudes towards disability and towards men and women with disabilities becoming parents. Disability, sex and sexuality have, in the social imagination, been problematic.

Disability and sex

The idea that women (and men) with disabilities might have sexual desires, have sex or reproduce has provoked dispute. It seems that the sexual identities of the disabled are particularly marginalized. As Buurman (1997) illustrates with images of the disabled as 'erotic bodies', the disabled woman is a sexual one too. The need to provide positive role models for the disabled parent is exemplified by the project Parentability, supported by the National Childbirth Trust and described in Chapter 8. The claim being made is that disabled women and men are capable and entitled to become parents. Sexual performance – that is, how disabled people have sex, has been defined as a medical problem, and therefore regulated, and to an extent legitimated by, medical discourse. However, the social acceptability of a disabled woman reproducing, especially where hereditary conditions might be passed on, or where they are deemed incapable of caring for a child, continues to be questioned. Disabled women report being denied adequate support, counselling and health care on issues of sexuality, birth control and fertility and are often encouraged to be sterilized (Lonsdale 1990; Asch and Fine 1997).

Women with disabilities are particularly disadvantaged because, in the view of men, they are more likely to be regarded as both physically and sexually unattractive and are frequently treated as asexual (Lonsdale 1990). Asch and Fine (1997) suggest that evidence from the USA indicates disabled women are less often (compared with disabled men and able-bodied women) successful in attracting a mate, and less likely to be in a heterosexual relationship. In the UK, women with disabilities and of working age are more likely to be divorced or separated than men with disabilities or other women (Lonsdale 1990). The stereotypes and images of disabled women are predominately negative and as a result they are excluded from the areas of social life normally open to women – nurturance and reproduction. Disability is socially produced, not reducible to bodily impairment (Oliver 1990) (see Box 6.5). In the nursing literature there is recognition that social attitudes towards disability and sexuality lead to **social exclusion**. But the solutions proposed are counselling for disabled people, and **social integration** to provide more 'sexual opportunities' for them. The

> **Box 6.5   A social model of disability**
>
> 'Disabled people' are not the problem – disability is the effects of:
>
> • Stereotyping – negative social attitudes towards disabled people as impaired and dependent on others.
> • Discrimination – caused by ableist attitudes: assumptions that being able-bodied is 'normal' which underpin the way society is organized, for example the view that only able-bodied women may care for a child.
> • Disadvantage – lack of access to well-paid jobs, housing, education and health care.
> • Social exclusion, isolation and segregation.
>
> *Sources*: see Saranga (1998); Lonsdale (1990); Oliver (1990).

focus is the disabled person rather than a change in health care practitioners' negative behaviour and attitudes (Morgan 1994).

Assumptions about a woman's ability to nurture and care for either a man or a child make a woman with disabilities undesirable for a man:

> Disabled persons (men and women) often elicit in non-disabled others powerful existential anxieties about their own helplessness, needs and dependencies (Hahn 1983). For a man who may have such emotional residues well-buried, their activism in the presence of a disabled woman may stimulate reflexively his rejection of her. Even if a man believed that a particular disabled woman could manage to run her own life and master the details of helping him with his, how could he accept help from an unwhole, 'sick' woman? . . . If men fear both their own and another's dependency and intimacy to the extent that Chodorow (1978) and Gilligan (1982) have argued, if disabled persons awaken such feelings, and if men desire women who can satiate their own emotional needs without either publicly acknowledging them or requiring reciprocity, disabled women are likely to be rejected forcefully as lovers/partners.
>
> (Asch and Fine 1997: 245)

Such undesirablity would no doubt be compounded by any question about the woman's ability to engage in penetrative sex. In addition, disabled women have been subjected to sexual abuse and exploitation by male carers and family members (Lonsdale 1990; Asch and Fine 1997). Such experiences contribute, in Asch and Fine's account, to problems in identity formation and the achievement of a culturally valued feminine identity. Although a disabled woman may have a more positive identity, the choices open to this group are constrained by negative attitudes towards disability, sexuality and reproduction. As a result these women are less likely to become mothers.

Contraceptive use and being child-free

For many women the ability to control their own fertility means greater control over their lives. Contraceptive technology and legalized abortion have been instrumental in facilitating this. However, this ability has both advantages and disadvantages as already implied above. Sex without fear of pregnancy means that sexual pleasure can be separated from reproduction. Abortion and the use of contraceptives have created other health problems for women.

Contraceptive technologies have themselves been associated with increased health risks and according to many feminists have been designed primarily with the sexual interests of men in mind (Doyal 1995). The increased responsibility placed on women to control their own fertility, following the development of contraceptive technology, has been regarded as reinforcing male power. As Doyal (1995) discusses, heterosex is more risky for women than sex between women. Heterosex can, and often does, have detrimental psychological and physical effects on a woman's health. Risks of HIV infection and venereal disease are significant for women but those who want also to become pregnant cannot protect themselves against HIV or venereal disease because 'babies and condoms do not go together' (Doyal 1995: 84). All women are at risk of HIV infection but Doyal's point is that heterosexual women are at greater risk than lesbians (see Richardson 1993b, 1996b; Waldby 1996 for a fuller discussion of these issues). Reproductive sex is hazardous, not least because pregnancy and motherhood can mean 'unsafe sex'.

Being child-free is however an option for many women today though the social pressures to become a mother may be intense (see Chapter 5). But the availability of contraceptives and other health services is related to public policies which themselves may be seen as reinforcing heterosexist ideologies and perpetuating views of women's sexual identity as tied to both reproduction and motherhood. The statistics on sterilization which 'is now the most popular method worldwide for preventing pregnancy' (Doyal 1995: 106) point to widespread sexism. Although male sterilization is cheaper and technically easier an estimated '70 per cent of all sterilisations are performed on women' (Doyal 1995: 106). The preferred intervention is on women's bodies, even though this is a more complicated procedure and is associated with more health risks. However, those women who are lesbian, or those who are involuntarily childless, do not necessarily choose to remain child-free.

Lesbian sex and motherhood

Lesbian women, as discussed in Chapter 7, are frequently denied the opportunity to become mothers using assisted conception techniques because they do not fulfil the (social) condition of sex with a man. Such policies and practices reveal the ways in which these technologies are culturally produced and socially contingent. Lesbian groups have therefore developed their own support networks and advice on how to conceive a child through self-insemination (Saffron 1994) and other health issues (Wilton 1997).

However, there are differences of view within lesbian groups about the significance of becoming a mother. While some lesbian women see motherhood as a creative and positive step, others see it as contradictory to being a lesbian because they reject traditional roles for women and a biologically driven destiny (Walton 1994). My view is that seen in this way, the links between sex, gender and sexuality become conflated again and such criticisms mirror a form of heterosexist thinking and biological determinism.

Widespread opposition to lesbians becoming mothers characterizes homophobic attitudes among health care professionals and government. As Wilton (1997) argues, lesbian mothers are seen as 'mad, bad or dangerous to know' and there is hostility towards them. Legislation and policy measures have been introduced which discriminate against lesbian women who want to become mothers, denying them access to fertility treatments, adoption and fostering opportunities as well as health care that recognizes their particular needs (Stern 1993; Walton 1994; Wilton 1997).

Involuntary childlessness

By contrast those heterosexual women who are involuntarily childless may be encouraged to seek infertility treatments in order to fulfil their socially expected function as mothers. Debates about the value of such treatments therefore frequently centre around the unnecessary tying together of a feminine sexual identity with motherhood and the passionate desire of the involuntary childless woman to bear a child (Pfeffer 1993). Those women with 'reproductive impairment' are disabled since 'despite major changes in the nature of women's lives, the status of "mother" continues in most cultures to be a central element in the definition of a "normal" adult female' (Doyal 1995: 146). The desire for a child is therefore understandable, yet those who suggest a woman is less of a woman if she does not (or cannot) reproduce draw on a specific and limited concept of gender identity. Only mothers, according to such a view, are 'real' or complete women (see Chapter 5).

As Symonds and Hunt (1996) suggest, a rigid definition of femininity and motherhood implies 'either lesbianism is part of being a "natural" woman or motherhood is not' (p. 119). This neither allows for the possibility of 'real' women choosing not to become mothers, unless perhaps they are lesbian, or lesbian women choosing motherhood.

Infertility treatment

As I shall discuss in Chapter 7, the new reproductive technologies themselves are shaped according to dominant norms of heterosexist culture. Pfeffer (1993) argues that the focus on women's bodies during treatment of infertile couples, even where the male partner may be in some way 'dysfunctional', reinforces sexist thinking and certain ideas of masculinity and femininity. The responsibility to reproduce is primarily the woman's. Doyal (1995: 147) argues that 'infertility can be a major disability and

> **Box 6.6 Researching assisted conception**
>
> In a study of women undergoing IVF treatment, Sarah Franklin (1997) describes the process as a series of 'obstacles' they had to overcome. She sees their experiences of treatment as 'a way of life' and describes the central part it played in their own, and others', view of their selves.
>
> In her discussion of the media coverage of 'success' stories infertile couples were consistently portrayed as 'desperate' for a child. The desire for a child was naturalized as part of the 'natural' life cycle that included marriage and parenthood. For the women themselves, infertility was experienced as disruptive of what was natural and many talked about feelings of inadequacy, lack of fulfilment and failure, even when their partners had been identified as 'at fault'. At the same time though Franklin describes how going through IVF treatment was for some women a means of making something of themselves, an achievement, and gave them a sense of purpose. Although failure was common this served to reinforce the need to try again and to keep at it. The 'choice' to have IVF treatment was paradoxical in these accounts, both a choice and one that was made *for* the woman who 'had to try' since they wanted a child. Moreover, the belief that a woman, by undergoing IVF treatment, has 'tried everything' turns out to be unfounded since IVF always presents the possibility of continuing with treatment or having another go, which Franklin suggests can lead to feelings of 'desperateness'. It is not therefore that women are desperate necessarily to have a child when they start treatment, but that the treatment itself contributes to the production of 'desperateness'. Franklin argues that IVF may be seen to fuse together science and nature as embodied progress.
>
> *Source:* Franklin (1997).

its treatment should be seen as a basic element in reproductive self-determination, along with abortion, contraception and maternity care'. Yet the experiences of infertile women are diverse across nations and social divisions. Some are more able to access services and treatment than others. This is sometimes related to the costs involved, but also to the assessment criteria used to select women 'suitable' for treatment (Doyal 1987; Walton 1994; Wilton 1997). Research into the experiences of women seeking assisted conception highlights the pressures they face (see Box 6.6).

From the discussion so far we see how sex and reproduction are tied together in heterosexist culture and how they are also frequently linked, even today, to marriage (Chapter 5). Therefore both lone (unmarried, divorced, separated and widowed) or child-free women and lesbian women, in different ways, represent a threat to the social order, and so too do infertile women. Unmarried or single women in particular may be seen as a threat to those who are married, since they offer the potential of sexual activity outside marriage. Child-free women represent a failure or refusal to engage in procreative or reproductive sex. Lesbian women, by rejecting heterosex, are often expected to give up any rights to motherhood. Those women who are infertile are regarded as incomplete and failed women, sometimes by themselves as well as many others. By decoupling sex and reproduction these groups of women may be seen in a more positive light and the specificities of their sexuality more fully understood.

There is, then, no inherent contradiction or connection between being a lesbian woman and being a mother or between being an heterosexual woman and not having children. Neither is there a justification for believing that only able-bodied women should become pregnant or give birth. One key reason why these groups of women are frequently consigned to the margins and socially excluded is because sex and reproduction (and marriage) are repeatedly tied together.

Conclusions

In this chapter I have discussed sexual identities and how they are produced. In particular I have argued that we need to rethink the links between sex, gender and sexuality. We need to see identities as fluid and changing and resist the tendency to naturalize them, to categorize and position individuals according to their sex, gender or sexuality. In reality, identities are produced through the intersection of discourses, institutions and bodies. The significance attached to different types of bodies is socially and historically contingent. Sexual difference cannot simply be reduced to biological differences, 'sex' cannot simply be understood in terms of biology. Rather, the patterning of sexual behaviour and the ways in which differences are brought into view is through the disciplinary and regulatory effects of discourses and social institutions. Medical, nursing and midwifery discourses are all implicated in this process as constructing relationships of power. Nature and culture are not separate spheres – what appears 'natural' or 'normal' is a culturally mediated product.

Health care provision needs therefore to take account of diversity, to meet the needs of different groups and recognize how identities are produced. At the same time the ways in which health policies themselves reinforce social division and inequality needs to be considered. For example, contraceptives, abortion and infertility treatments should be available to those who may engage in a variety of sexual practices. We need to avoid reinforcing heterosexist ideologies or making moralistic assumptions about what is normal or deviant. Rather than preventing marginal groups such as lesbian women from access to those services which enable them to control their own reproductive lives, we need to examine ways to include them. At the same time the targeting of services, or directing of them towards specific groups, needs to take account of how such measures act as a means of social control and a disciplinary force.

Sex is not simply about reproduction but about desire and pleasure. The regulation and disciplining of desire is socially accomplished. Sexual health and maternity services play a part in regulating sexual behaviour and reproductive choices. What is needed is a reflexive awareness of the part such institutions play, the ways they reproduce medical and moral discourses about socially acceptable behaviour and limit the 'choices' available to people. Being a woman is not necessarily about being a mother (and neither is being a man necessarily about being a father). At the same time, being lesbian or homosexual need not preclude the possibility of becoming a mother or father. Those men and women who are involuntarily childless, or those who choose to be child-free, need not be regarded as inadequate or nonconformist. They need services made available to them that they regard as appropriate. Similarly the sexual health and reproductive lives of disabled women and men could be enhanced by recognizing the frequent discrimination which occurs when normative assumptions about disability and sexuality are made. What I hope this chapter has shown is that a sociological perspective on the organization and regulation of sexuality, sexual behaviour and sexual identities offers important insights into how health services may be improved.

Summary

- This chapter considered the importance of understanding sexuality for health care practice. I described the ways in which identities are produced and the relationship between identity and the body. Crucially this means understanding the connections between the biological and the social. Rather than seeing bodies as biological givens, biological 'sex' was seen as discursively produced.

- The categorization of different types of bodies as 'male' and 'female' was seen as historical and tied to the development of modern society.

- The processes of civilization, rationalization and secularization were linked to the rise of scientific knowledge and medical discourse. Scientific approaches to the body and sexual behaviour characterized the modern era.

- The effect of these theories was to shape social attitudes and public policy towards sexual practices.

- Women's sexuality has for a long time been seen as problematic but so too have homosexuality, teenage sexuality and disability and sexuality.

- Heterosex – that is, sex between men and women – has been regarded as the norm, and was institutionalized within marriage. Moreover sex and reproduction were tied together and non-procreative sex was considered deviant and immoral.

- The organization of sexuality relates to relationships of power and inequality. The construction of 'difference' results in social division and discrimination.

- By rethinking the links between sex, gender and sexuality we can begin to see the effects of discrimination and heterosexism. This in turn could enable health care practitioners to improve their practice by considering how best to meet the needs of diverse groups.

Discussion points

- What is hetereosexism?
- How do we explain the organization of sexuality in modern society?
- In what ways have sex, reproduction and marriage been tied together?
- Why has it been suggested that we need to loosen the links between sex, gender and sexuality?
- What are contemporary attitudes towards lesbian women and homosexual men becoming parents?
- What influences health policies regarding the use of contraceptives, abortion and infertility treatments?

Further reading

Connell, R. (1995) *Masculinities*. Cambridge: Polity Press.

Franklin, S. (1997) *Embodied Progress: A Cultural Account of Assisted Conception*. London: Routledge.

Hawkes, G. (1996) *A Sociology of Sex and Sexuality*. Buckingham: Open University Press.

Petchesky, R. (1986). *Abortion and Woman's Choice, The State, Sexuality and Reproductive Freedom*. London: Verso.

Saranga, E. (ed.) (1998) *Embodying the Social: Constructions of Difference*. London: Routledge.

Walton, I. (1994) *Sexuality and Motherhood*. Oxford: Butterworth-Heinemann.

Wilton, T. (1997) *Good for You: A Handbook on Lesbian Health and Wellbeing*. London: Cassell.

Woodward, K. (ed.) (1997) *Identity and Difference*. London: Sage.

PART 4

WOMEN'S BODIES

REPRODUCTIVE TECHNOLOGIES AND THE NEW GENETICS

Introduction

In the preceding discussion about how identities are socially constructed I have highlighted how the relationship between bodies and identity has been problematized. Rather than seeing a direct relationship between them, the ways in which bodies are typified as male and female was seen as historical and characteristic of a modernist society. Recognition of the contingent formation of identities also means rethinking what it means to be a body, or to have a body. In drawing together both social and biological aspects of being I have suggested that this has implications for how we think about reproduction and mothering. I have argued that the links between sex and reproduction may be seen as a product of heterosexist thinking which emphasizes particular kinds of social and sexual relations.

In this chapter I turn to the debates surrounding the development of new reproductive technologies (NRTs) and the new genetics. Here we shall see that women's bodies are viewed in contrasting ways. Debate may be characterized as a continuing controversy about the connections between biological and social processes and how these are mediated, or produced, by technological innovation. My view is that these technologies are at the same time constructed by, and produce, social relations.

Reproductive technologies are big news, the human story, the ethical and legal issues sell newspapers and have been the subject of numerous television programmes. Headlines such as 'Can a widow be a mother?' (*Guardian* 1996), 'Cell-by date for embryos' (Burdet 1996) and 'Woman could die bearing octuplets' (Dillner 1996b) all highlight increasingly complex decisions surrounding the development of these technologies. They mark out an area of vigorous public debate that has focused attention on reproduction. Writing in the early 1980s about the advent of artificial reproduction (now also referred to as assisted reproduction) with the birth of the world's first 'test-tube baby' in 1978, Oakley described it as 'the most fictional, and yet, now real, scientific scenario of all' (Oakley 1986: 281).

Eighteen years later Dillner, writing in the *Guardian*, said 'it is not surprising that people worry that medicine has built the technology without the ethical scaffolding' (Dillner 1996a). According to her, a chance remark by an obstetrician and gynaecologist saying that a woman wanted to have a twin pregnancy 'downsized' by having one of the foetuses removed revealed 'a gap between what doctors think is normal practice and what the rest of the world thinks' (Dillner 1996a). Dillner points to a lack of information about such practices and a continuing patchy provision of teaching in ethics for medical students. So what has been going on in the past 18 years? What in Oakley's terms is this 'new world of scientifically engineered parenthood' (Oakley 1986: 282)? What kinds of questions might we ask about these developments? According to Oakley there are two central ones: first, is assisted reproduction a good thing?; second, who controls the new reproductive technologies?

More recently it has been suggested that we need to ask different kinds of questions and that the debate around NRTs may be characterized by two approaches: fundamentalism and liberalism (Farquhar 1996). A third way proposed by Farquhar reframes the debate and suggests that we need to rethink the relationship between these technologies, women's bodies and their social identities.

Drawing on the earlier work of feminists in this area (see for example Arditti *et al.* 1984; Corea 1985; Stanworth 1987; Spallone 1989; McNeil *et al.* 1990; Stacey 1992; Rowland 1993), in the first section, I shall outline the fundamentalist view of these technologies. These writers draw on feminist criticisms of scientific knowledge and the medicalization of women's lives. This will lead to a discussion of whether technology can be seen as neutral. In the second section I develop an analysis of women as subjects and explore liberal discourses of 'rights' and 'choices'. I then consider how these technologies destabilize conventional notions of women as mothers, men as fathers, and families, and consider the idea that NRTs dissolve and fragment 'woman' as a unitary identity. Finally, I shall focus on the new genetics and developments in genetic services, and consider what kinds of reproductive choices women are faced with since the growth of genetic testing and screening.

Technological innovation

Spallone (1989: 14) provides a useful definition of NRTs:

> The term *new reproductive technologies* (NRTs) is recent. The NRTs include IVF, embryo transfer, sex preselection, genetic engineering of embryos, cloning (making genetically identical individuals) and more. They are new because they are relatively recent developments, based on new capabilities. But they come from the scientific approach to reproduction which brought us the 'old' reproductive technologies such as hormonal contraceptives (the Pill) in the 1950s and the 60s and pre-natal screening (amniocentesis) by the late 1960s. Reproductive technologies, old and new, include genetic technologies.

The development of NRTs is chronicled in the reports of the scientists behind them, medical practitioners, social scientists and newspapers. A large number of feminist writers have been strongly critical of them while others have supported their use (Arditti *et al.* 1984; Corea 1985; Stanworth 1987; Klein 1989; McNeil *et al.* 1990; Rowland 1993). Many of these accounts begin with the story of the first 'test-tube baby', Louise Brown, born in 1978, though as Spallone (1989) describes, the research techniques were being tried out in the years preceding this event. She outlines the early work of IVF pioneer Robert Edwards as originating in his research in the 1950s when he first became interested in IVF in mammals. Accordingly, the new reproductive technologies may be seen as an expansion of earlier animal research and the growing science of genetics. Spallone (1989: 84) suggests, in a compelling way, that these scientists continue to 'use women as experimental material for laboratory research into reproduction', and that the failure to trial new techniques or conduct research using primates (because they were too time-consuming) marked a particular attitude to women and women's bodies. She says, 'contrary to popular understanding, IVF experimentation on women's body parts was being carried out *alongside* animal experimentation, before the methods were established in other mammals' (Spallone 1989: 89, original emphasis).

Careful analysis of the careers and work of individual scientists such as Edwards and Pincus, Rock and Chang (who developed the Pill) reveals, in Spallone's account, their primary interests in scientific knowledge and technological development. For these scientists technological advances and the pursuit of scientific knowledge were motivating factors in setting their research agenda and organizing research activities, rather than any concern with women's health. The early development of the contraceptive Pill as a method of regulating and controlling women's fertility can be seen as closely tied-in to pharmaceutical company interests and population control. The fertility of women is construed as a 'problem' in social policy (see Chapter 6). For *pronatalists* the problem is to encourage women

Table 7.1 IVF treatments: live birth rates

Live birth rate – per embryo transfer	18.3%
Live birth rate – per egg collection	16.7%
Live birth rate – per cycle started	15.1%
No. of patients treated	23,153
Total treatment cycles	30,216
Stimulated treatment cycles*	24,182
Singleton births	3,201
Twin births	1,247
Triplet births	161

* Note that these are figures to indicate where a woman's ovaries have been stimulated to produce more than one egg per cycle.

Table 7.2 IVF treatments with donated eggs or embryos

Treatment with donated eggs or embryos	
Cycles with donated eggs	1,110
Cycles with donated embryos	216
No. of live births	243

Table 7.3 IVF treatments: frozen embryo transfers

Frozen embryos	
Frozen embryo transfers	4,908
No. of live births	580

to have more babies (of the right kind), while for *antenatalists* the problem is to restrict and limit women's capacity to reproduce (Pfeffer 1993). Spallone argues that 'IVF and hormonal contraceptives are two sides of the same reproductive technology coin' (Spallone 1989: 89). Chemical control of ovulation is often part of the IVF treatment programme.

Links between research scientists and medical practitioners are crucial in both securing the necessary 'raw material' for research purposes and trialling experimental techniques. Hence the famous partnership of Edwards and Steptoe – the obstetrician who delivered Louise Brown. The raw material, as Rowland (1993), Spallone and other feminist writers point out, is women's body parts and they emphasize the **commodification** of body parts in their accounts. So women in clinical settings are seen as 'living laboratories', the experimental subjects of laboratory research: 'Women in clinical settings have been the experimental subjects of IVF researchers as surely as a female rabbit sitting on their laboratory benches' (Spallone 1989: 90).

Despite these criticisms the data shown in Tables 7.1–7.4 give some idea of the current use of NRTs and the activities of 101 DI (donor insemination) and IVF clinics and 'storage centres' in the UK licensed to carry out

Table 7.4 Donor insemination treatments (excluding GIFT)

Live birth rate per treatment cycle started	9.2%
Patients treated	5,956
Total treatment cycles	16,659
Stimulated cycles	6,803
Singleton births	1,416
Twin births	118
Triplet births	12

Note: GIFT = Gamete Intra Fallopian Transfer (donor gametes). Fifty-four GIFT treatment cycles were carried out between the dates indicated above.

various treatments (HFEA 1997). All the data relates to the period between 1 April 1995 and 31 March 1996. It is clear that many women do use NRTs, though the effects are complex (see Chapter 6 and Pfeffer 1993; Franklin 1997) and the 'success' as measured by the live birth rate is low. Many 'treatments' therefore fail to produce a live child.

Salvation or damnation? A polarized debate

In their powerful and passionate critique of NRTs feminist writers have highlighted a number of important issues which lie at the centre of the debate surrounding NRT use. These issues are informed by wider feminist critiques of the nature of scientific knowledge and different views of women as subjects. Debate focuses on the extent to which these new technologies are beneficial to women or whether they are a particularly perverse form of oppression for women. Framing the debate in this way sets up a polarity between the idea that these technologies represent either a 'patriarchal victory' and conspiracy by medical men to control women (the fundamentalist argument), or a liberalization and greater freedom for women (the liberalist view). As Farquhar (1996) puts it such accounts situate NRTs in binary divide between 'salvation' or 'damnation'.

Spallone's (1989) analysis focuses on the status of science in the western world, and she asks whether technology can be seen as neutral. She, like other commentators, also draws attention to an opposition set up between the status of women and the status of embryos. In order to assess the validity of her analysis we need to develop an understanding of feminist critiques of scientific knowledge and different views of women as subjects, human agency and action.

Science in the western world

The *Human Fertilisation and Embryology Act* of 1990 (Department of Health 1990) provides the legal framework for the development and use of NRTs in the UK. It defines the meanings of terms such as 'embryo', 'gamete', 'mother' and 'father' (for a detailed discussion of human embryo research see Mulkay 1997). It amends the earlier *Surrogacy Arrangements Act* of 1985 and the abortion laws of 1967 and 1987 and has been influential in shaping policy at the European level. But, according to Spallone (1989), the scientists supporting IVF and Baroness Mary Warnock, the philosopher who chaired the select committee which recommended the terms of the Act, saw scientific 'facts' or biological 'facts' as neutral and given, but also providing the basis of ethical standards. Scientific rationality is seen by them, and many others, as the guiding principle for discussion of ethical issues. This, says Spallone, is tautological because the 'facts' are seen as the basis for deciding ethical questions which, in turn are to set the standards for scientific activities. The conclusion that she reaches seems a justifiable one – that 'IVF scientists seem to have it both ways, scientific knowledge is neutral (never bad) and science is positively good (never bad). By the science-is-neutral argument, science and technology remains "technical" and "value-free"' (Spallone 1989: 27). This points us towards a long-standing debate within the social sciences and philosophy about the claims of scientists and the **hegemony** of scientific rationality in the western world, and feminist criticisms of science as objective and value-free.

I have already discussed in Chapter 2 the ways in which the power of the medical profession has been based on claims to expert knowledge and scientific objectivity. Such claims have glossed over the effects of the medicalization of life and specifically the ways in which pregnancy and childbirth have been 'captured' within the remit of medicine as potentially risky and pathological processes (Oakley 1986). Here once again we see the relevance of understanding how scientists have accrued certain privileges based on their claim to be neutral and objective.

Historical analysis of the development of scientific endeavour identifies 'the rise of the age of science' from the Renaissance period and is briefly outlined by Gordon (1991). He describes the demarcation of science from religious belief and the secularization of science (see also Turner 1995). While the authority of the Church had until that time been the means by which truth and falsehood were determined, the claim to scientific knowledge was based on empirical evidence. Early scientists challenged the hierarchical order and authority of the Church and argued that reason, and the evidence of the senses, was the basis of scientific knowledge, and that this was accessible to everyone. Enlightened men (*sic*) were therefore 'free to use what reason they possess[ed], without subservience to authority' (Gordon 1991: 25). 'Scientific method' was seen as providing the means to understand the natural world. These early scientists believed that all men (*sic*) were rational beings, capable to a greater or lesser extent of using scientific methods, but they did not recognize that science itself created a hierarchical order. By making universal claims about scientific truths that they regarded as constant across cultures and independent of the status of the knower, they set scientific knowledge apart from other forms of knowledge and belief.

The social construction of scientific knowledge – a discursive practice

In his introduction to *Science, Technology and Society*, describing a visit to the Science Museum, Webster (1991: 1) notes that 'the authority of science relies precisely on our perceiving it as something that lies outside society: science is not, in these museums, a contested terrain, an arena where differences of opinion and division appear . . . Science deals with "facts"'.

This presentation of scientific 'facts' in the modern world has been an *ideological* achievement. While initially the age of science and triumph of reason was seen as divorced from the social and political relations of the time, more recently the intimate relationship between them has been made explicit in the work of various sociologists of science. The production of scientific knowledge began to be seen as the product of a social and political consensus (Kuhn 1970; Collins 1985; Webster 1991). By problematizing the status of scientific knowledge as in some way special and distinctive, some sociologists problematize the very idea of 'science'. According to Woolgar 'science' is seen as constituted by social relations and discursive practices. Woolgar (1988: 14) shows how 'The discourse of science is to be understood as a discourse which structures and sustains a particular *moral order* of relationships between agents of representation, technologies of representation and their represented "objects"' (my emphasis). According to this analysis the authority of science rests on an ideology of representation which claims a special status for scientific knowledge as 'factual' and true.

Feminist criticisms of science

Many feminist writers have argued that scientific knowledge is androcentric and sexist (see, for example, Harding 1986, 1991; Hekman 1990; Alcoff and Potter 1993; Stanley and Wise 1993; Rose 1994). They challenge the scientists' universalizing claims to objective, value-neutral knowledge and instead draw attention to the ways in which science has perpetuated the ideas of a dominant elite. These writers see knowledge production as a political process that systematically excludes the voices of women and other oppressed groups. As Hekman points out 'since the Enlightenment, knowledge has been defined in terms of "man", the subject, and espouses an epistemology that is radically homocentric' (Hekman 1990: 2). Feminist critiques of the development of NRTs draw on this view in order to show how the claims of scientists to be objective and value-free rest on the validity of scientific knowledge and their ability to gloss over the power relations that are embedded in their work.

In *Love, Power and Knowledge* Rose (1994) also outlines feminist critiques of science. According to her in the early days the focus of concern was the small numbers of women involved in scientific activity, and later the erasure of women such as Rosalind Franklin (whose work in crystallography is now acknowledged as crucial to the 'discovery' of DNA) from historical accounts of science. Subsequently there have been attempts to develop a feminist critique of epistemology drawing on the radical science movement and social studies of science. For these feminists, critiques of science as patriarchal begged the question of what could replace it – could there be a feminist science?

While there is disagreement among feminists about the answer to this question, and a range of positions on the issues (see, for example, Hekman

> **Box 7.1 A summary of some of the key criticisms made by feminists of 'masculinist' science**
>
> ● The claim to universal truth assumes that all knowers are the same – this ignores important (gender) differences between those that 'know'.
> ● The claim to objectivity assumes a distance between knower and the object of study and ignores how values and interests impact on the production of knowledge.
> ● Conventional empirical scientific methods (e.g. observation and measurement) applied to humans treats them as objects rather than knowing subjects.
> ● The emphasis on 'rationality' denies the importance of other experiential aspects of human existence such as emotions and embodiment.
> ● The making of generalized statements about women's lives ignores important differences between women.

1990; Harding 1991; Richter 1991; Tong 1992) it is possible to identify some of the criticisms that have been made of scientific knowledge (see Box 7.1).

Put simply, *Standpoint feminists* such as Harding (1986, 1991, 1993) argue that because of their particular standpoint in society, women are able to be more objective (that is, women do better science). Women, they say, are able to propose alternative truth claims based on a critical realist viewpoint and empiricism. According to this view, by recognizing their position in the world and the links between knowledge and social position, women are able to produce more accurate (objective) knowledge. ***Postmodern*** *feminists* are also critical of scientific knowledge but they do not argue for a strong view of women as knowing subjects (see, for example, Hekman 1990; Richter 1991; Tong 1992 for a discussion of this). Instead postmodernists highlight the ways in which both knowledge and subject positions are constructed through discourse (see also Chapter 8).

Is technology neutral?

Some feminist writers who support the development of NRTs do so on two counts: – first that the technologies themselves are benign and that in the right hands, that is in women's hands, they could be beneficial; second that these technologies extend women's right to choose when, and how they reproduce. Let us examine these ideas. The belief that if women had better or more control over the use of these technologies then many of the issues would be resolved assumes that technology is indeed neutral. That is to say the 'techniques' of IVF, AID (artificial insemination by donor sperm) and embryo lavage are potentially beneficial, but they are commonly in the wrong hands and out of the control of women. According to Farquhar (1996) the difficulty with both fundamentalist and liberal approaches to these technologies is that critics see technologies as fixed and as having an **ontology** of their own. Therefore the tendency is to see the effects of NRTs as overdetermined by the technology. Spallone (1989), who represents a fundamentalist position, rejects this argument saying that the logic of these technologies is to replace patriarchy with control by technocrats. She believes that eugenic, racist, sexist and ableist values are tied into the technologies which are neither neutral nor benign. The power relations between inventors and users of these technologies cannot, in her view, be liberating for women, as women are required as exchange body parts for 'progress'. Even without husbands (a feature of patriarchal society) women would be at the mercy of reproductive engineers. If women had positions of control it seems likely that some would be making eugenic decisions about which embryos to 'choose' and which 'genes' to perpetuate. Spallone says that although some might argue that these technologies could potentially subvert patriarchal structures of the nuclear family (by enabling women to have babies without husbands or sexual relations with men), new forms of subordination would be created where technocrats or 'experts' would have power over women.

In mapping the transition from small to 'big' science – the strengthened links between capital, government and scientific research – Rose (1994) sets the debate around NRTs in a 'transformed technoscience landscape'. Rose notes that 'While there has been an immense feminist literature studying, analysing, debating the new technologies, searching for a new politics, it has done so largely in a framework which rather rarely explicitly draws on theories of (science and) technology in society' (p. 175). Rose identifies three theoretical approaches that may usefully be woven together and argues that science and technology are intimately bound together and that there is no sense in separating them in any discussion of NRTs:

1 *Social constructionism*: as we have seen already social constructionists such as Woolgar (1988) emphasize that science is a product of what scientists do and say; that knowledge is constructed through the day-to-day activities of scientists which are organized around technological artefacts and networks of actors.
2 *Externalism*: this relates to the power relations which are reproduced by scientific knowledge so that the interests of powerful, elite groups are advanced through the production of knowledge which is classist, sexist and racist. Accordingly the power structures of society such as class, patriarchy and white supremacy are instrumental in shaping research activity and technological innovation.
3 *Technological determinism*: this is the belief that technology is autonomous and separate from society but shapes relationships around it.

So, says Rose (1994: 176), 'In the sense that the new reproductive technology feels as if it is pursuing its own unstoppable masculinist logic, strands within feminism share more than a little of this strong determinism'. She too is critical of the notion that the effects of NRTs are overdetermined by technology but she wants to see science and technology as intimately connected. The problem is that where feminists see science and technology as separate, according to Rose, this reproduces 'that ideo-logical binary split between science and technology – preserving the "purity" of science while admitting the "dirty" worldly nature of techno-logy' (Rose 1994: 176). She says this is a mistake, that technoscience and the development of NRTs must be understood as part of 'a dominant and global culture'.

So technology may not be seen as neutral after all, but it has no separate ontology and neither does science. Neither is it irretrievably corrupted or imprinted with inherent inequalities. Rather, if we follow Farquhar's view and that of other postmodern feminists (Haraway 1991; Sawicki 1991) the effects of NRTs are contradictory and sometimes unintentional (Farquhar 1996). Their argument is that rather than seeing the technologies as always only having negative or positive consequences, there is always the possibility of both. NRTs may be both controlling and liberating. While accepting that technology is mediated by social relations, the ways in which this happens is not fixed but dynamic and changing. Accordingly it is unhelp-ful to suggest that the effects of masculinist science are totalizing and overwhelming. This is a pessimist and dystopic view. Instead Farquhar (1996) suggests that fundamentalists are inherently conservative in their approach to NRTs drawing on, and reinforcing, fixed (essentialist) and unchanging concepts of technology, 'woman' and 'families'. In contrast it is precisely the destabilizing effects of NRTs that, Farquhar argues, presents the possibility of their reappropriation by women to advantage and benefit. The next section therefore examines the consequences of NRTs for con-ceptualizing 'women' as subjects in a liberal democracy where their voices have frequently been ignored.

Women as subjects

Feminist critiques of science, and more specifically NRTs, have been underpinned by a concern that women have disappeared from view in the language and practices of research scientists, clinical practitioners and policy makers. It has been argued that research activities which have rendered women as experimental subjects, test-tubes or laboratories, and simultaneously given embryos a status outside women's bodies, have sig-nificantly undermined the status and subject position of women. For, in so far as the new technologies have encouraged the view that IVF and other techniques are dependent on technological expertise and know-how, women's bodies have been both devalued and written out of the picture. The notion that life, in embryonic form, may be sustained outside a woman's body transgresses previously accepted and understood boundaries. At the same time, the invasive approach of techniques such as egg collection, embryo lavage and insertion of drugs, instruments and other technical paraphernalia crosses boundaries in both directions by entering into a woman's body and taking parts away. It is for this reason that critics such as Spallone (1989) argue that technology cannot be seen as neutral, for it configures the user in certain ways. She claims that particular views of a woman's body are deeply embedded within the technologies themselves.

The writings of Rowland (1993), Arditti *et al.* (1984) and Spallone (1989) make serious and important points about the effects of reducing women to laboratories or test-tubes. However they are criticized for being fundamentalist because they appear to adopt an essentialist view of women and women's bodies (see Chapters 6 and 8). In their discussion of women's rights and whether women have a right to choose these technologies they draw on a liberal and modernist conception of the humanist subject (see Chapter 8). This raises additional questions about how far the liberal discourse of rights and choices is appropriate for understanding and advancing feminist projects.

Liberal discourse of rights

There is tension between the notion that women have reproductive rights and should be able to 'choose' when to become pregnant, and how to give birth. Recognizing some of the difficulties Spallone (1989: 83) says, 'The concepts "reproductive rights" and "reproductive choice" have been co-opted by medical science and other agents of the state to advocate medical/scientist controlled, technological reproduction'. She suggests that we need to reassert our rights and examine how choices are limited: 'The most important questions for women are why are we given *some* "choices" and not others, and why are certain women allowed to decide among a particular set of reproductive options, while other women are not?' (p. 83, original emphasis). Spallone refers to Rowland's (1993) suggestion that for feminists the 'right to choose' is better understood as our demand for the 'right to control' our own bodies. Forty per cent of women who 'chose' surrogacy in a study by Winslade (1981), reported by Spallone, were unemployed or on welfare benefits. Poor, black women from Mexico or Central America were regarded as useful and acceptable for gestating embryos created with eggs from white women in North America (see Arditti *et al.* 1984; Corea 1985). These examples suggest that the conditions under which women make 'choices' are often coercive and oppressive.

Betterton (1996), in her discussion of assisted reproductive technology, asks whether a woman's right to choose should extend to choosing the genetic identity of her baby. She outlines the debate like this:

> For feminist critics like Gena Corea, the association of terms like 'choice' and 'freedom' with the new technologies is a perversion of feminist rhetoric, used to justify scientific experiments over which women themselves have no control. Rachel Bowlby reframes the debate in more useful terms when she asks how far a liberal discourse of rights and choice is appropriate to the area of reproduction at all.
>
> (Betterton 1996: 116)

For Betterton, and Bowlby (1993) 'choice' relates to consumer behaviour in the free market and has superseded earlier notions of civil or human rights, 'and as with other areas of consumer choice, new technology opens up possibilities for which it then creates both needs and desires' (Betterton

1996: 116). Betterton therefore draws attention to the ways in which 'choices' are socially constructed, how new services create new demands and new technologies extend market possibilities. For Bowlby then, rather than seeing this debate in terms of agency versus victimization, or choice versus imposition, we need a more thorough analysis of the desires and identifications people have of themselves as mothers, or not. According to Bowlby we should not assume as given that the wish for a child is either natural or a right (see Chapter 5). Certainly we need to ask how the market in maternity services, and development of genetic screening is being shaped and how this influences the 'choices' women make. In addition we need to think through what kind of liberal democratic model underpins these accounts.

As Spallone (1989) and others point out, embedded in the policies and legislative framework of the UK is a continuing reliance on a definition of personhood that is universal and undifferentiated. So we find: 'In the name of equality Warnock rendered "his" and "her" gamete donation the same, rhetorically masking with abstraction the more than slight difference between masturbating into a glass and having surgery' (Rose 1994: 181). Moreover, the Warnock committee defines the personness of the embryo as beginning after the fourteenth day (Warnock 1985). Prior to this, research is not seen as violating legal or ethical principles relating to human life (for a discussion of the later debate around embryo research leading to the *Human Fertilisation and Embryology Act* 1990, see Mulkay 1997). The committee drew on a universalist ethical discourse which is abstracted from specific historical, social and political relations, rendering both bodies and subject positions as invisible.

Gender differences

Another aspect of this debate on rights and gender differences is put forward by O'Brien (1981). She posits that while maternity is fundamentally a social dyad between mother and child, in contrast, paternity becomes social historically. According to her analysis fathers 'choose' how, and whether, to nurture and choose paternity by claiming rights to the child. Men, given their biological separation from their seed and the child, are only able to appropriate the child with the cooperation (consent) of others. O'Brien draws attention to the way in which, despite a universalist discourse of liberal rights where everyone is positioned equally, able to claim and exercise rights, there is a fundamental asymmetry between men and women with respect to paternity and maternity.

Bordo (1995) makes a related point showing how, under the law, the integrity of a man's body is maintained in ways that are not similarly applied to pregnant women. So, for example, while a man's right not to donate bone marrow to save his cousin's life was upheld by the courts in the USA, a woman's right to decide to have an abortion, or not to be sterilized has been overturned by the courts. In these cases a woman's right to decide has been rejected on the grounds that she is either an unfit mother, uncaring or evil, and that the rights and interests of the foetus should take precedence over hers. This, says Bordo, shows unequal rights for men and women with respect to the issue of informed consent for surgical or medical intervention. In the UK this has been brought sharply into focus with a recent controversy over whether a woman should be allowed to use the sperm of her dead husband to impregnate herself (Dyer *et al.* 1996). In this case, initially the UK Licensing Authority upheld the husband's rights and ownership of his body parts by refusing her permission on the grounds that he did not give his written consent – so the bodily integrity of the dead man was upheld. Subsequently the woman obtained the sperm and went abroad for treatment that enabled her to become pregnant (see HFEA 1997; HEFA 1995; also www.hfea.gov.uk).

In questions of fathers' rights to a child or unborn foetus it seems that the assertion of paternal rights is at the expense of maternal ones. Bordo (1995) argues that in the USA, though fathers claim equal rights when suing their pregnant partners to prevent an abortion, in such cases the rights of one must prevail over the other. Though sometimes the fact that the woman must bear the child has prevailed, in others the woman has been seen simply as an incubator for the baby and of little significance. In contrast, Shanley (1995) seems to suggest that rights should be tied to social relationships, not biology; that once a child is born, where a father can demonstrate he is a carer (or potential carer) his rights should equal the mother's. Therefore, according to this view, the biological connection of the woman to the foetus also assumes a reduced significance as the social role of parent is emphasized. This also opens up a space for surrogacy and the rights of surrogate mothers based on a biological role would similarly be weakened.

What follows therefore is that while a man may choose to claim (property) rights over his child, a woman has no such rights. For, in the debate around the viability of the foetus and the acceptability of research or clinical manipulation on embryos, the rights of the embryo are set in opposition to the woman. The effect of IVF has been to promote the view that women's rights are circumscribed by those of the embryo/unborn child. The interests of the unborn child are the primary consideration. The law thereby intrudes into the woman's body, crossing boundaries that have no parallels in the reproductive rights of men.

So while rights in liberal discourse are assumed to be universal and applied equally to men and women, it seems that in relation to reproductive rights asymmetries persist. In some accounts this is justified by mobilizing a form of biological essentialism which emphasizes the natural and biological role of women as childbearers and highlights sexual differences. However, in other situations the personhood of the foetus, and rights assigned to the unborn child, take precedence over those of the mother whose behaviour is deemed unnatural and violating her primary biological function to reproduce. A woman's right to choose is therefore constrained by dominant orthodoxies about what a fit and caring mother *should* do. Where feminists argue for a woman's right to choose to have infertility treatment and claim that the NRTs offer the possibility of liberating the infertile woman, they draw on this discourse of rights which asserts a liberal view of the human subject. In a sense they mobilize the essentialist and naturalistic concept of a woman as reproducer.

Destabilizing the subject

However, at the same time, postmodern feminists such as Farquhar (1996) and Shildrick (1997) highlight how these technologies destabilize concepts of the human subject. Relationships such as 'mother', 'father' and kin are revealed as unstable and socially constructed because, with the assistance of these technologies, reproduction may take place outside women's bodies, *in vitro*, or in the body of another woman. In this respect women's relationship to reproduction has been seen as more like that of men (Farquhar 1996). As men are separated from their sperm, so too may women become separated from their ova. Identities of mother and father therefore become fragmented into genetic mother, birth mother, surrogate mother, legal mother, and cannot simply be regarded as naturalized or reducible to biology.

For example, 'fatherhood' or being a father is constituted in a number of ways:

- 'Father' may be seen as a *biological* relationship, as the sperm donor or genetic father.
- 'Father' is constituted as a *legal* relationship when the birth of a child is registered or a child is adopted.
- 'Father' describes a *social* relationship.

Though these dimensions may interrelate, they are distinctive and should not be conflated together. In the context of NRTs the biological relationship of 'father' (or mother) is by no means a straightforward one. O'Brien (1981) noted that a man's relationship to biological reproduction is unlike that of the woman. The man is separated from his sperm and cannot be certain that he is the biological father of a particular child. This physical separation is emphasized by the sperm donor who gives his sperm with no expectation that he will come to know the child or care for them. In this sense sexual activity (masturbation in the case of the donor) is only indirectly related to reproduction for men. The heterosexual woman usually has greater knowledge of who the father of her child is for she is more able to know with whom she has had intercourse. But AID and IVF can have the effect of separating the woman from reproduction in similar ways to men (Farquhar 1996).

Today, both in the UK and USA, it is still the birth mother who names the father on the birth registration certificate, if she chooses. Registration of the father sets up the legal obligation and responsibilities of that man for that child. Such a system of legitimation of the child in effect legitimizes the father. Paternity rights and responsibilities are contingent on this legitimation process and, according to feminist writers, support a particular social structure (McRae 1993; Callahan 1995; Shanley 1995) (see Chapter 5). The extent to which legal paternity is linked either to the biological or the social relationship of father is variable. Legal debate about the position of surrogate mothers, birth mothers and social mothers highlights the contentious effects of the new technologies but also serves to demonstrate the social contingency of what were previously assumed to be 'natural' relationships.

Traditionally it has been marriage that conferred paternity on men and all children born in wedlock were legitimate. In contrast the illegitimate child had in the past to struggle to establish a legal relationship to its father or any claim against the father's estate (Smart 1987). More recently, Smart argues, there appear to be two directions in which the law has moved to support the idea of a heterosexual nuclear family. Where the biological father is most likely to provide this, the law reinforces his rights and authority. In other cases where the biological father is 'unsuitable' or unavailable, the law ignores the biological link. The primary consideration seems to be to underpin a particular social structure where the social father or head of household (for example the father of an adopted child, or a stepfather relationship) is responsible for the child. In the UK, following the 1989 Children's Act, there has been a continuing debate about the financial responsibilities of 'absent' or 'feckless' fathers. This debate has especially related to the work of the Child Support Agency (Westwood 1996) and highlights the reluctance of the state to support women independently caring for children. So the law works to reconstitute families (Smart 1987) even as reproduction becomes possible outside the confines of heterosex (see Chapter 6). Increased 'choice' may be linked to a commodification of health and maternity care, but the possibility of recuperating NRTs to benefit women is of value (Franklin 1997). The effects of the technologies are not one way and may, perhaps unintentionally, offer some women (and men) the chance of improving their lives.

Genetic screening and genetic testing

The development of NRTs includes the growth of the 'new genetics'. The Human Genome Mapping Project is the international research project to map the entire human genetic sequence and to identify genetic causes of ill-health and disease. This development may be seen as a new form of 'political interventionism': 'a product of the alliance between an aggressively entrepreneurial culture and the life sciences, fused with the conservatism of biology as destiny with the modernist philosophy of genetic manipulation' (Rose 1994: 173). Rose refers to the 'genetic turn' which marks a widespread and dramatic shift in biological politics. She says 'political interventionism' marks the attempt to push back the frontiers of science and technology in order to control and manipulate the basic unit of life. Genes are increasingly commodified in a political economy where bodies and body parts, especially those of women, are part of a broader process of the commodification of nature and knowledge. At the centre of Rose's analysis is the view that venture capital (private investment) has underpinned biological research since the 1970s and has backed the development of both NRTs and clinical genetics. In this final section I want to examine how the theoretical issues identified above have relevance to current policy making and the shaping of genetic and maternity services. Women's 'choices' have become increasingly complex and are made more so when presented with information now provided by prenatal screening and genetic screening.

Table 7.5 Current screening programmes available

Population group	Current available screening: condition and method
Antenatal pregnant women	Amniocentesis, chorionic villa sampling, rubella, Rh+/−, cystic fibrosis, neural tube defects, Down's syndrome, ultrasound
Neonatal	PKU, cystic fibrosis, sickle cell, congenital hypothyroidism, duchene muscular dystrophy, physical examination
Older children	Health screening, pilot genetic screening
Pre-conception adults	Cystic fibrosis, Tay-Sachs, haemoglobinopathies, colorectal cancer, breast cancer

Source: Adapted from Nuffield Council on Bioethics *Genetic Screening: Ethical Issues* (1993).

First I need to distinguish between different kinds of testing and screening. The Nuffield Council on Bioethics (1993) makes a distinction between *genetic testing* (testing an individual showing signs of a genetic disease/ condition) and *genetic screening* (a mass screening programme of a population). They also distinguish between the screening programmes of different populations (see Table 7.5).

Included within the term 'genetic screening' are different types of tests: those which directly identify genes/chromosomes linked to disease or abnormality; indirect tests which detect biochemical changes associated with genetic disorders; and physical examination or ultrasound, which visualize 'abnormalities' associated with genetic disease. Importantly for our discussion some genetic diseases are inherited while others are not (e.g. Down's syndrome is not inherited but a genetic mutation occurs; Tay-Sachs disease is an inherited disorder). So the eradication of all genetic disease is an unrealistic aim since there will always be mutations which occur. The cause of these mutations is often not the focus of attention and neither, it seems, is the link with environmental factors.

In discussions about developing genetic services and maternal welfare policies an entire vocabulary is built around the genetic status of individuals and groups. Some are 'affected', others are 'carriers'; moreover, the relationships between individuals and within 'families' become a focus of attention. As the Nuffield Council on Bioethics (1993) points out, individuals with no history of illness or disease may discover they are 'carriers' and be asked to consider the dangers of passing on a particular gene to another individual. And, the discovery of genetic information about one individual may have considerable implications for the genetic status of another related individual. While pilot screening programmes have been set up with research funding, the development of mass screening programmes is a subject of continuing policy debate.

The arguments in favour of large-scale screening programmes are founded on principles of promoting 'a health care system that aims to help people maintain good health as well as treating disease and accidents' (Nuffield Council on Bioethics 1993: 3). But genetic screening was regarded differently by the Council because the health of those being screened may not be directly at risk. Rather, genetic screening raises numerous questions about the responsibilities of individuals and governments towards each other. In weighing up the potential benefits against the potential harm of genetic screening, the Council suggested that it could identify treatable diseases at an early stage, give *couples* a chance to make informed reproductive choices, and eventually identify genetic susceptibility to common diseases that could be prevented or minimized. Set against this, it could increase anxiety for individuals and families, create difficult decisions regarding termination of pregnancies and have adverse effects on job opportunities and insurance ratings (McGleenan 1998). The Council pointed to the diversity of factors affecting the desirability and acceptability of genetic screening programmes and the wide range of opinion on this matter. However, they concluded by making recommendations with respect to information-giving and informed consent, results and confidentiality, employment, insurance, public policy and the implementation of screening programmes. Three years later the debate in the House of Commons continued. There was evidence that the insurance industry was proving reluctant to develop guidelines on the use of genetic information, and the efficacy of the regulatory role of the Licensing Authority was being called into question (*Hansard* 1996). The Human Genetics Advisory Commission was set up by the government in 1996 to advise on these issues and 'to advise on ways to build public confidence in, and understanding of, the new genetics' (Department of Trade and Industry 1997, www.dti.gov.uk/hgac).

Among critics, the central concerns remain as to whether these technologies, and the introduction of screening programmes, are sexist, ableist or racist. Is clinical genetics a form of eugenics or non-directive counselling; big business or health promotion; health for all or survival of the fittest? In so far as genetic research uses and abuses women and women's bodies, it is sexist. If the pressures to produce 'perfect babies' leads to a continuing neglect and erosion of rights and resources for disabled people then genetic screening is ableist. Where genetic disease is racialized and leads to discrimination against specific 'racial' groups or where the intention is to clean up the gene pool or genetic stock of a group, it is racist.

Researching genetic services

Clinical genetics is at the centre of controversies surrounding the application of new genetic knowledge. The implications of this new knowledge for clinical practice are being widely discussed though Weatherall (1991) argues that the ethical issues and problems identified are not fundamentally new ones – rather, they are extensions of existing clinical practice. He points out that genetic screening and prenatal diagnosis have been accepted procedures for many years. However, he acknowledges public concerns that clinical genetics may be a form of eugenics (the effect he says of ignorance and media hype), and that it is sensitive because there is a danger of stigmatization and personal concern about carrying 'bad genes'. He suggests a number of measures that would assist in making clinical practice acceptable. Drawing on experiences in the USA, and with reference to a few studies looking at genetic screening programmes, Weatherall emphasizes the importance of well-designed screening programmes based on small-scale pilot studies. For him 'the great importance of preceding a population screening programme by a period of intense education at all levels of the community' (Weatherall 1991: 351) needs underlining for it is essential for the success of the programme. In his view, education and promoting the public understanding of science will lead the public to recognize the 'rational' and 'logical' basis of genetic research and screening. In addition, genetic counselling will reduce the psychological stress and negative effects of screening. He suggests that 'ethnic minority groups are particularly sensitive' and the UK experience of introducing prenatal diagnosis of thalasseamia in London demonstrates the importance of an 'adequate education' to prepare communities for screening. Weatherall dismisses debate about embryo research as 'emotional and often illogical' and is encouraged by the passing of legislation (Department of Health 1989a, 1990) which indicates that 'reason has prevailed'. At the same time however, good clinical practice is seen as an art, and genetic counsellors as crucial in the delivery of effective genetic services.

From this account it becomes evident that while scientific rationality is seen as the basis on which legislation and government policy should be formulated, the application of this in clinical practice relies on the effective communication skills of individual practitioners and the education of potential clients or patients. The importance of teaching medical students both the science (molecular biology) and the art (communication) of clinical practice has indeed become a focus of attention (Royal College of Physicians 1989). Research into the delivery of genetic services has also been prioritized (Rogal College of Physicians 1990; MRC Initiative 1994; Health Technology Assessment 1995; DoH 1995). So far a number of completed studies highlight the effects of going for genetic screening, the importance of training for health care professionals, and factors affecting the uptake of testing.

Studies of the psychological effects of prenatal testing and serum screening have looked at levels of anxiety and attitudes to the pregnancy. A study of serum testing for Down's syndrome showed that women who receive a positive test result experience considerable anxiety (Green 1990; Statham and Green 1993) but that the reasons for undergoing the test in the first place influence a woman's response to it. Some saw amniocentesis as part of 'intelligent prenatal care and expected a benign outcome', while others who had a history of 'affected' children were more anxious and saw such tests 'as part of a relentless process challenging what was previously believed to be a normal pregnancy' (Green 1994: 40). Different types of test – diagnostic tests rather than screening (the former identifies *whether* the baby is affected, the latter identifies the *risk* of the baby being affected) also have different effects. Attachment to the baby has been seen to increase after a negative test result has been received, highlighting the contingency and tentativeness of pregnancy created by such tests (Katz Rothman 1994). Other studies suggest that where serum screening for neural tube defects is routine in certain hospitals and the result is normal, it does not create anxiety but neither does it allay anxiety (Green 1994). Abnormal results however do create anxiety, as do false positive results (those that turn out later to be normal).

Green's (1994) discussion of these studies leads her to conclude that women's reaction to screening and the psychological effects must be understood within a broad social context in addition to the specific circumstances of the individual test. The routinization of screening tests seems to reduce their significance for individuals but the predictive power of screening tests is poorly understood by both health care staff and patients (see also Davison *et al.* 1994). Green advocates increased social support (genetic counselling) for women and better information for both groups (Statham and Green 1993). But what is also needed is a sociological analysis, which goes beyond the psychological and examines the ways in which health behaviour and use (including issues of access) of health services are socially constrained and shaped. There is also a need to reconsider the effects of professional power and medical discourse. Medicine has powerful ideological effects in shaping the understandings women have of what their experience of pregnancy should be, and how 'responsible' women should act.

Agency and control

Prenatal tests such as amniocentesis, chorionic villus testing, ultrasonography and genetic screening reinforce the idea that it is both natural and a right to want a perfect baby (Chadwick 1990). But this is contentious (see Box 7.2). 'In the names of prevention and prediction, coercive practices are increasingly being introduced' (Rose 1994: 191). Screening programmes which in effect offer only a choice about whether to go ahead with a pregnancy where risk of 'abnormality' is high and a judgement about whether, given poor public services for disabled people, parents could cope, are unacceptably coercive, says Rose (1994: 193). She argues that a political ploy of those favouring genetic screening is to talk up serious conditions where few women would choose to go ahead (e.g. Huntington's disease) and transfer this to other forms of genetic impairment without acknowledging complexity.

So, according to Rose, in cases where, for example, Huntington's chorea is diagnosed, for which there is no known cure, genetic screening may be seen as presenting a new dilemma: *uncertainty + hope* or *certainty + no hope* (1994: 195). Similarly, Katz Rothman (1994) says genetic testing lets us think we can replace chance with choice. However, Davison *et al.* (1994) believe that there is a widely-held misconception about the certainty of genetic information (see also Richards 1993). As Rose suggests, we need to see the impetus for these services against a background of international cooperation and the Human Genome Mapping Project. Government and commercial agencies are central in advancing this work, setting the research agenda and developing policy on the provision of services. And, as already argued, although women are seldom represented in these fora they are central to the work, in so far as their body parts are necessary for research.

Women are drawn into increasingly complex decisions through the application of these technologies. Moreover these decisions are individualized and the experience of pregnancy becomes 'tentative' (Katz Rothman

> **Box 7.2 Researching genetic counselling**
>
> Recent research and writing in the area of genetic counselling raises fundamental issues about the ways in which agency and control are exercised in reproductive decisions.
>
> - First there are questions about how far counselling can be non-directive (see Clarke 1991; Clarke, 1994; Abramsky 1994).
> - Research on the effects of prenatal tests on a woman's psychological well-being shows that women who test positive for Down's syndrome become very anxious (Green 1990; Statham and Green 1993) but different tests have different effects (Green 1994).
> - The fact that some tests are seen as 'routine' obscures both the arguments for pre-test counselling and the possibility of non-directive counselling (Marteau et al. 1992). As Abramsky (1994) points out, the very act of 'offering' a test presupposes that such a test is both desirable and morally acceptable.
> - The provision of pre-test counselling as part of antenatal care has been described as patchy, unclear and poorly presented. Although Abramsky (1994: 83) suggests that 'this is not a cause for despair' but reason to 'think how we can improve it', it seems that there is cause for alarm.
> - The consequences of such practice are that women are ill-informed and poorly supported, making decisions to terminate pregnancies on partial or poorly understood information and enduring both physical and psychological suffering (Statham 1994).

1994). No longer are women encouraged to feel confident or assured of their ability to reproduce. The burden of responsibility for 'congenital abnormality' and 'deformity' is placed firmly with the pregnant woman, while the environmental, social, political and material conditions which give rise to genetic mutation or disease, and its disabling effects, are conveniently swept aside. The decision about whether to give birth to a child with a disability is seen as a personal one with personal consequences (can she cope?) rather than a collective social responsibility. Eradicating deformity is prioritized over changing social attitudes or promoting a caring society (Hubbard 1997). In certain respects we can see this as flowing from a rights perspective where the individual autonomy of women is asserted through the right to choose.

This emphasis on reproductive decision making presupposes that the woman is an autonomous individual who will make the right (rational) decision. Given the right information, in the correct way, a woman is expected to be able to judge for herself what is the appropriate course of action. But the literature on prenatal screening and therapeutic abortion suggests that rationality and logic are not the best indicators of what it is like for a woman to terminate a pregnancy (Statham 1994). In *The Tentative Pregnancy*, Katz Rothman (1994: 2) believes that 'The new technology of reproduction encourages and reinforces the commodification process, genetic counselling serves the function of quality control and the wrongful life suits are a form of product liability litigation'.

The emotional and experiential aspects of pregnancy are, according to Katz Rothman, undervalued (and undertheorized). For, at the same time as being expected to care for, and love, her unborn child, the pregnant woman is expected to be able, and willing, to abort the foetus if it is found to be 'damaged'. On the one hand the personness of the child is invoked as deserving of care and love while on the other, the foetus is objectified as damaged and unwanted. When the pregnancy reaches 24 weeks the child will be protected by the law as a person, but contradictorily, abortion for 'handicap' negatively identifies 'the damaged foetus' beyond this time.

The importance of 'expert knowledge'

There are, then, a number of theoretical problems that run through the literature. The establishment of a genetic link seriously weakens the concept of the autonomous individual, central to liberal theory (Rose 1994: 195). This is evidenced by the repeated concerns that families are the real subjects of clinical genetics (Richards 1993). Indeed to hear geneticists talk of their 'family trees' gives a clear indication of how individuals become subsumed within their genetic heritage, a heritage appropriated by others. Again, while the notion of agency rests on some concept of (relative) autonomy, in the context of clinical genetics the individual becomes dependent on the interpretation of clinical data and family trees by expert clinicians or counsellors, and is incorporated into an area of professional practice. Experiential knowledge of one's own body is seriously undermined as new knowledge on the molecular level is presented. The slogan 'Genes R Us' emphasizes this. Even while questions of identity may be thrown up (Who and what am I?), when being asked to take responsibility for one's own decisions the individual is drawn into a professional discourse and ideology about what it is important to know. The technology, the science, this new knowledge, creates a new set of questions about where to locate oneself and how to reassess the experiences of the past. Measuring this previous self-knowledge against the professional and scientific expertise presented in a counselling session is indeed likely to be difficult.

People who choose not to know, or do not take up the offer of screening are portrayed as in need of education. This 'deficit model' has been used to justify a large-scale education programme to develop public understanding of science (Department of Health 1989a; Weatherall, 1991; Nuffield Council on Bioethics 1993; Levitt 1998), and genetic literacy (Turney 1995) so that the public may appreciate the value and importance of scientific, genetic knowledge. If mass screening is to be associated with mass education and the training of health care workers to disseminate genetic information and provide counselling, this represents a significant and costly objective for the NHS. It also has the potential effect of extending the sphere of influence of professional/medical power and expert systems of knowledge at a time when the legitimacy of both has been increasingly questioned in the context of a modern 'risk' society (Beck 1992; Giddens 1991). So the new genetics may represent a more extensive colonization of human life by medical and scientific discourse. However, many women resist screening programmes, refusing to attend or take advice. Weatherall (1991) reports that 17 per cent of a sample of graduates said they would not accept the offer of amniocentesis in pregnancy to screen for Down's syndrome. This indicates that the effects of these discourses are not totalizing and both lay and expert accounts of genetics coexist. The 'deficit model' undervalues the knowledge and 'expertise' of lay persons (Kerr *et al.* 1997, 1998).

Towards a feminist ethic?

Surrounding these debates on the merits or acceptability of genetic screening programmes is a growing literature on professional ethics (Chadwick 1990; Clarke 1994; Koehn 1994). Professional philosophers have sought to explore the ethical issues and present guidelines for professional practice. Rose describes the 'institutionalization of ethics' as a liberal democratic response to social criticism of science with an ethic of no ethics (1994: 180) and the rise of bioethics as sidestepping issues of professional and masculinist dominance. In her view ethicists may even have given a new gloss to professional power. Professional ethics depoliticizes the issues and recasts them as technical problems. Criticisms of the Warnock Committee, outlined above, seem to bear this out. And even where consultation with lay organizations has taken place the role of the experts and the weight attached to scientific evidence favours professional and masculinist values (Dunkerley and Glasner 1998).

Shickle and Chadwick (1994) propose 'a modified utilitarian approach' to making decisions about which kind of screening programmes should be made available. Such a view attempts to draw up a balance sheet of costs and benefits and 'a trade-off between the harm brought about by screening and the harm brought about by failure to screen' (Shickle and Chadwick 1994: 15). Recognizing that 'providing a screening service may give the counsellee the impression that the "correct choice" of action would be to accept screening' (p. 16) Shickle and Chadwick argue that obtaining 'informed consent' does not remove responsibility for harm from those who offer the screening. For Shickle and Chadwick the criteria for offering screening is that the majority of the population would accept it. Shickle and Chadwick believe that individual patients cannot be objective about ranking their needs; that involving society is time-consuming, expensive and over complex. Consequently, 'we see little alternative to the existing decision-making process, provided that this is in consultation with experts and lay organisations. We recognise that this will be biased by the social values of those involved' (p. 17). So Shickle and Chadwick advocate *majoritarian* rule and the role of experts is secured. Their model offers no analysis of the representativeness of lay organizations such as the Genetic Interest Group (GIG 1998) or the power of experts. The bias and subjectivities of individual patients are swept aside even though the social values of professionals and lay organizations are acceptable. Justice is conceived of in terms of procedures which make screening available to all, though rationing is inevitable and justified.

My interest is how a feminist ethic of care might also inform this debate (see Chapter 4). Within a liberal humanist framework, first the connections of the woman and embryo can be seen as fundamental, as in accounts like Spallone's (1989, 1992) above. Second, mutual dependence rather than autonomous/possessive individualism would characterize the feminine subject. Related to this, responsibility and obligations, care for the other, and taking the view of the other leads to a view of reproductive decisions which relates to both the subjective wishes of the individual woman and her assessment of the benefits or harm to her unborn child. In this view, the child has no status separate from the mother. This implies that rights are not to be seen as oppositional or a zero sum, but *interdependent*. The rights of one are not at the expense of the other. Reproductive decisions informed by an ethic of care include the need for others to be obligated to care. So it is not just a question of the individual preferences of a woman – the obligations of others (society) to care for her and her baby whether or not it is perfect need to be taken into account.

Conclusions

NRTs and the new genetics may be seen as both controlling and potentially liberating. My concern is that, in the context of a society still riddled with social division and inequities, women will not easily be able to turn these technologies to their actual advantage. Therefore while there is the possibility of subverting or resisting dominant discourses around NRTs, in practice this proves very difficult. At the same time the focus on genetic disease, screening and artificial reproduction could enable us to address important and pressing concerns about why women want to be mothers, the expectations we have of motherhood, attitudes to disability and deformity, and links between the environment and health.

In my view, the status of women as subjects and citizens appears to be weakened, rather than enhanced, by these technologies while at the same time we are held responsible for making reproductive decisions that will benefit the wider community. This doesn't seem empowering – rather, it appears to isolate and individualize the pregnant woman. Pregnancy is still seen by many as a natural given for women but also increasingly as something they should do *well*. The experiential and emotional aspects of pregnancy are frequently lost in a debate about what is ethical, rational, logical and acceptable to society. The search for greater control, greater certainty or even perfection creates a situation where it is hard for any woman to know what to do or feel. Instead failure and uncertainty somehow seem more likely. Women who terminate a pregnancy due to foetal handicap do not talk of being victors and women who undergo infertility treatment do not always describe a positive experience (Franklin 1997). Evidently, like most things, NRTs and the new genetics have the potential for good and for harm, and as women our relationships to them are likely to be ambivalent, contingent and complex.

Summary

- In this chapter I have attempted to review the debates surrounding the development of NRTs and genetic screening services. I have done so by examining the relationship between science, technology and women's bodies. Sociological perspectives on this have been drawn from the social studies of science and feminism.

- A great deal has been written on this subject but following Farquhar (1996) I identifed three main approaches to the issues: liberalism, fundamentalism and postmodernism.

- The key issues identified were the status of science in the modern world and the links between science and technology. Science was seen as 'masculinist' and feminist criticisms of science were briefly outlined.

- I then discussed the extent to which NRTs are neutral and whether they configure a particular set of social and political relationships. The claim by some feminists that women have been used as experimental subjects and their bodies abused is a substantial one. But these technologies may be seen as having both intended and unintended consequences. Therefore they are not themselves fixed or static, but culturally mediated in ways which make the reappropriation and recuperation of them a possibility.

- Liberal and fundamentalist approaches to the technologies may be seen as naturalizing and essentializing 'women', assuming that they all stand in a similar relationship to the technologies. At the same time these analyses portray the effects of medico-scientific discourses as totalizing and overdetermined by the technologies.

- In contrast, a postmodern discourse-analytic approach points to the ways in which the technologies rupture and destabilize identities of 'mother' and 'father', crossing bodily boundaries. This presents the prospect of reconfiguring 'women', of enabling them to find diverse ways of using these technologies to their advantage.

- NRTs and the new genetic technologies are both constructed by and constitutive of social relationships. They are neither all bad, nor all good – rather, their effects relate to the ways in which social processes interact with them.

Discussion points

- Do NRTs represent scientific progress?
- How far do women benefit from NRTs?
- What are the implications of these technologies for women as subjects?
- What kinds of choices are available to women and to what extent do they control their own reproductive lives?

- What evidence is there that genetic screening programmes are sexist, ableist or racist?

- How do women experience prenatal screening and genetic counselling?

Further reading

Callahan, J. (ed.) (1995) *Reproduction, Ethics and the Law: Feminist Perspectives.* Bloomington, IN: Indiana Press.

Farquhar, D. (1996) *The Other Machine: Discourse and Reproductive Technologies.* London: Routledge.

Franklin, S. (1997) *Embodied Progress: A Cultural Account of Assisted Conception.* London: Routledge.

Katz Rothman, B. (1994) *The Tentative Pregnancy: Amniocentesis and the Sexual Politics of Motherhood.* London: Pandora.

Pfeffer, N. (1993) *The Stork and the Syringe: A Political History of Reproductive Medicine.* Cambridge: Polity Press.

Rose, H. (1994) *Love, Power and Knowledge: Towards a Feminist Transformation of the Sciences.* Cambridge: Polity Press.

Stacey, M. (ed.) (1992) *Changing Human Reproduction: Social Science Perspectives.* London: Sage.

EIGHT

IMAGING BODIES

Introduction

This chapter explores in more depth what it means to have a body, to be a body and more specifically to be pregnant and give birth. It also examines how representations of bodies produce meanings that shape our understanding. What a body is, and how we understand the significance of bodily changes, is not straightforward. At a common-sense level we may think we know that bodies have certain physical characteristics and are essentially biological organisms that breathe, eat, move, sleep and think. Though there has, historically, been a tendency to universalize bodies, to see them as more or less similar, actually this tells us very little about what a body is or about specifically female bodily experiences such as pregnancy and childbirth. It also tells us very little about differences between bodies. In Chapter 2 I described two models of pregnancy and childbirth, the medical model and the midwifery model. The differences between these two models were characterized by different methodologies; different ways of knowing. Medical knowledge emphasized scientific methods of inquiry and treatment while the midwives emphasized experiential and practical knowledge as important for midwifery care. Here I want to consider how these two models conceptualize the body and more specifically, women's bodies.

In certain respects we can see that both doctors and midwives think about women's bodies in similar ways. The universalizing discourse of science, used by doctors, treats bodies as more or less the same and operates within a set of normative definitions about how healthy bodies look and function. These ideas and theories are invoked to justify the medical management of pregnancy and clinical intervention. Midwives frequently describe pregnancy as a 'normal' and 'natural' process which, because it is natural, does not require medical intervention. However, the 'naturalness' of women's bodies is taken for granted.

As I argued in Chapter 6, differences between women and their diverse relationships to their bodies are often ignored and, like the doctors, midwives may be seen as treating women as an homogeneous group. So, though midwives are often critical of medical science by emphasizing sexual differences between male and female bodies, and by claiming pregnancy is a 'natural' event, they rest their case for a midwifery model of care on a form of biological essentialism. Naturalizing women's bodies in this way is, from a sociological point of view, deeply problematic.

As I indicated in Chapter 1, the body has become of central importance in social theory. Davis (1997: 1) describes the embody-ing of theory and explains that:

> different explanations have been put forth for this recent 'body craze'. For some, the concern is regarded as a reflection of the culture at large. Others view the current interest in the body primarily as a theoretical development. And, for still others, feminism is held responsible for putting the body on the intellectual map.

She points out that for feminists, research on the body has been a focus for many years (see also Bordo 1995). Much of this research has looked at issues around reproduction, including menstruation, pregnancy, abortion, infertility, NRTs and menopause (Martin 1993; Darke 1996). While this research has sought to draw attention to the importance of these aspects of women's lives there has developed a long-standing and continuing debate about how we conceptualize women's bodies. This debate has centred on the extent to which nature and culture intersect and the relative significance of each of these.

In this chapter I shall develop some of the ideas discussed in Chapters 6 and 7. In discussing the formation of sexual identities I explained that the connections between sex, gender and sexuality are not straightforward. While some feminists highlighted gender differences, the extent to which these were related to sex differences was seen as contentious. The binary division between 'men' and 'women' was seen as an historical one, a feature of the modern western world. Increasingly this gender divide has been criticized as obscuring other differences between women, and between men, and for ignoring similarities between men and women. For example, the marginalization of black women or lesbian women, working-class or homosexual men, remained unexamined. Therefore the concept of 'gender' has been questioned and the sexing of bodies seen as arbitrary (Butler 1993; Gatens 1996).

In the first section I will consider why the recent emphasis on embodiment has been seen as bringing bodies back, as highlighting the lived experiences of being and having a body. The body has always been seen as a site of domination and oppression by feminists who 'focused on how women's bodies have been regulated, colonised, mutilated or violated [and] in the wake of the "linguistic turn", the focus in feminist theory on the body shifted from women's experience of oppression to how images of the female body were implicated in power relations' (Davis 1997: 10–11). However, Davis suggests that this focus on domination has underplayed the agency of women – the ways they resist power or subvert efforts to control them. Through embodied practices Davis and others argue that transgression is possible, that women are active in shaping their own lives through daily practices. Queer theory, constructionism and cultural critique suggest ways to disrupt power relations.

In the second section I look at images of women's pregnant bodies in art and popular culture to see how power is exercised through these. Drawing on art and cultural theory I show how the external appearance of the pregnant body has been constructed as a sealed vessel, an object to be looked upon. I will explore how medicine visualizes women's bodies and the development of new ways of seeing using diagnostic imaging. During pregnancy, visualizing inside the woman's body has helped create the foetus as a new subject for medicine and, as suggested in Chapter 7, erased the woman as subject.

Finally, I consider the implications of seeing the inside and outside of a woman's body as connected and continuous. The boundaries of inside and outside are seen as blurred and a feminist view of 'leaky' bodies emphasizes this feminine subjectivity (Shildrik 1997). As I shall explain, this view of pregnant bodies is potentially disruptive because it undermines the notion of a modernist subject. Following Young (1984), the notion of a maternal subject is problematic and the work of women artists and photographers highlights the possibility of subversion and transgression. So while the focus of this discussion is the representation of pregnancy my intention is to link together the symbolic and the material, to see pregnancy and childbirth as having both a materiality and symbolic significance, to be embodied practices.

Theorizing bodies

Historically, as we saw in Chapter 6, it has been argued that women are equated with or stand for nature, that which is natural, emotional, uncontrollable and chaotic (Turner 1992) while men have represented culture,

the rational, controlled and controlling force. Dualism and dichotomous thinking has divided men/women along lines of mind/body and in
effect women have been reduced to their bodies (Bordo 1995). Haraway
(1991) and others have argued that the division between nature and culture is a capitalist and patriarchal one, a product of a particular historical
period and that the development of the biological and social sciences
reproduced this division. Paradoxically and controversially then, those
feminist critics who have argued for a revalorization of women's bodily
experiences have been seen as reinforcing, rather than undermining this
dualism (Annandale and Clarke 1996). Emphasizing the differences between
male and female bodies may be seen as essentializing those differences,
treating them as if they were natural. Such a view also tends to gloss over
the differences between women and, like the midwives above, treats all
women the same.

In contrast, arguments for recognizing that gender is socially constructed
and that the sexing of bodies is a cultural process have opposed essentialist accounts with constructivist ones. Constructivists focus on the social
and cultural processes that construct men and women as distinct groups.
Differences are seen as socially produced, rather than being 'natural' or
biologically determined, as we saw in Chapter 6. The opposition between
these two positions has been criticized by Fuss (1989) who suggests that
they are not really oppositions at all but that each depends on, or presupposes the other. Moreover to say there are differences between 'men' and
'women', male and female bodies, is not necessarily to say these differences are fixed or immutable (Gatens 1996; see also Chapter 6). So there is
no simple polarity here between essentialist and constructivist accounts
even though it is frequently presented in this way. Rather, as we shall see,
the material and the symbolic meanings of the body are both important.

Materiality and representation

In a discussion of feminist theory and the sociology of human reproduction Annandale and Clarke (1996) argue that modernist feminists and
postmodern feminists conceptualize women and women's bodies in contrasting ways. The former emphasize gender differences but while 'liberal
feminists argue there is no intrinsic relationship between sex/biology and
gender . . . radical feminism takes a contrasting view which endorses a strong
connection between sex and gender' (Annandale and Clarke 1996: 20).

The subject 'women' is central to these modernist analyses. According
to them the **poststructuralist** or postmodern approach is best characterized by a focus 'on how subjectivity is shaped, not on how individuals
shape the world' (Linstead 1993 cited in Annandale and Clarke 1996: 21).
A poststructuralist approach therefore **deconstructs** gender and a binary
opposition between 'men' and 'women' is undermined, as we saw in
Chapter 6. Annandale and Clarke are however criticized for undermining the work of midwives and feminists who have improved the care of
pregnant and parturient women and for in effect 'rehabilitating technological obstetrics' by suggesting that some women find technological control of childbirth 'liberating' (Farquhar 1996; Campbell and Porter 1997).

Moreover, their proposal that cyborg imagery represents a radical challenge to modernist ideas of science/technology as 'simply male demonology' is seen as a potentially dangerous way of conceptualizing personhood in so far as it reconfigures women as machinery rather than human subjects (Campbell and Porter 1997). Haraway (1991) discusses the cyborg myth as a way of thinking about a postmodern political subjectivity which transcends the boundaries of human and machine, enabling creative possibilities for a future where there is no gender, where identities are not unitary and bodies are not seen as bounded. Of course, in their defence of modernist feminisms Campbell and Porter re-mobilize the concept of the human subject and re-emphasize the physical suffering and pain of women. What is at issue here is the relationship between sex and gender and how the 'subject woman' is conceptualized, but also women's embodied experiences of pregnancy and childbirth.

Central to this debate is the relationship between the material body and how it is represented. Materiality refers to the material, corporeal and physical presence of a body. Bodily presence is the site of action and according to some commentators the foundation of knowledge (Stanley and Wise 1993). The symbolic refers to what the body signifies, how it is represented and what meanings it carries or produces. Thus, bodies have both a material and physical reality and symbolic significance though much research in the past has emphasized *either* the materiality of the body *or* culturally produced representations. Increasingly, the relationship between these two aspects has been seen as important, both to embody theory and to understand how bodily experience is culturally mediated and discursively produced.

Materialist feminisms

In the last chapter my discussion of NRTs examined the work mainly of materialist feminists (modernists) who were critical of the treatment of women in the development of these technologies and their use. Spallone (1989) and other radical feminists focused on the ways in which women's bodies were dismembered and highlighted the coercive exercise of power by medical scientists and physicians. They may be seen as extending other criticisms made of how maternity services have been medicalized and the ways in which women have been 'captured' (Oakley 1986). Materialist feminism sees the body as 'gripped' by culture and focuses on how women's bodies are shaped by power (Bordo 1995). This is a politics of the body (Jacobus *et al.* 1990). However, Davis (1997: 8) suggests that 'feminist theory concentrated on the cultural meanings attached to the body or the social consequences of gender rather than how individuals interacted with and through their bodies'. According to her, while the distinction between sex (nature/the biological) and gender (culture/the social) was useful for feminists it meant that bodies remained undertheorized, seen as underpinning cultural representations, a 'backdrop' to culture. So materialist feminists have been criticized for taking biological sex differences for granted and for not going far enough in analysing *how* nature and culture intersect in their discussions of gender.

Postmodern feminism(s)

Postmodern feminists focus on the processes of social construction, as I discussed in Chapter 6. The emphasis of these accounts is the symbolic, the ways bodies are discursively produced or fabricated (Shildrik 1997). Following Foucault, power is seen as productive and constitutive, not simply acting upon bodies but creating and shaping them. Critics of such an approach argue that the materiality of the body is neglected – it is as if biology does not matter at all, and in particular the fact that bodies are produced from *women's* bodies is overlooked (McNay 1992). The focus on disciplinary power and the regulation of bodies has been criticized as a form of cultural determinism. Individuals may be seen as relatively passive, as disembodied, rather than embodied, active and reflexive. This is much disputed, and the idea of resistance is important for seeing bodies as a site of struggle, where discourses compete, or intersect, shaping individuals and being shaped by them. Butler's (1993) argument that 'sex', rather than being a biological given, must be seen as a normative and discursive category which produces the materiality of the body therefore deconstructs gender and loosens the link between sex and gender, as we saw in Chapter 6.

Embodied practices

While feminist debate may be characterized as a division between modernist (materialist) and postmodernist (poststructuralist) projects, increasingly there has been a recognition that the lessons learnt from each need to be integrated:

> bodies are not simply abstractions, however, but are embedded in the immediacies of everyday, lived experience. Embodied theory requires interaction between theories about the body and analyses of the particularities of embodied experiences and practices. It needs to explicitly tackle the relationship between the symbolic and the material, between representations of the body and embodiment as experiences or social practice in concrete, social, cultural and historical contexts.
>
> (Davis 1997: 15)

So, bodies may be seen as combining the symbolic and material, mediating both biological and social processes (Darke and Kent, forthcoming). Frank (1991a) suggests we see bodies as constituted within a triangle of discourses, institutions and corporeality. He argues for a view of the body as process 'not an entity but the process of its own being' (p. 96). Shilling puts it another way saying the body 'is unfinished at birth, an entity which changes and develops throughout an individual's life' (Shilling 1993: 100). For him the idea of the body as a project conveys the sense of dynamic interaction between the organic (material) body and social processes (see also Shilling 1997). Turner (1992) makes a distinction between having a body, doing a body and being a body. However, theorizing bodies from a feminist perspective requires analysis of how, in the process of embodiment, power differentiates bodies from each other, marking them as different and materializing those differences. So for example the work of feminists such as Young (1990), Bordo (1995) and Davis (1997) is important for showing how the feminine body is produced and lived; how 'feminine' embodiment is accomplished.

The implications of seeing bodies as unfinished projects or a process are both theoretical and methodological:

- At the methodological level a **phenomenological** approach emphasizes lived bodily *experiences* (Young 1984, 1990; Frank 1991b, 1996).
- Institutional analysis focuses on the ways in which particular social *institutions* such as the state, the health service, the labour market and the family shape health and illness (Doyal 1995).
- A discourse analytic or cultural analysis approach focuses on the *representation* of bodies in literature, science and popular culture (Bonner *et al.* 1992; Martin 1993; Adams 1994).

Though each of these may be seen as connected and interrelated, the level of analysis tends to emphasize different aspects. For this reason critics suggest that in discourse analysis the materiality of the body is neglected, and that phenomenological approaches underplay the importance of social institutions in structuring individuals' experiences. Institutional analysis can appear to gloss over the discursive aspects and imply that such structures are immutable (fixed) and constituted separately from either bodies or discourses. The difficulty in theorizing bodies is tied to a methodological debate about how we know what it is to have a body and to be a body, and what it means to be pregnant or give birth. Although we may see these different levels of analysis as interlinked, each methodological approach offers useful insights that help us to understand how pregnancy and childbirth are socially constructed, embodied practices. Recognizing the connections between nature and culture points to the importance of analysing how culture produces bodies.

Representation

In an excellent discussion of representation Hall (1997a: 2) explains that '*Culture*, it is argued, is not so much a set of things – novels and paintings or TV programmes and comics – as a process, a set of *practices*'. Language may be seen as a representational or signifying practice whereby meanings are produced using words, pictures, music and other symbols. We use these practices to describe bodily experiences and to produce knowledge about those experiences – for example, by telling stories about pregnancy and birth (Oakley 1979; Adams 1994; O'Connor 1995). The women in Oakley's (1979) study described feelings of agony and ecstasy associated with birth. These mixed feelings tied together pain and joy, disgust and pleasure, excitement and fear. Childbirth was seen as a trauma and a drama, sometimes as an achievement (a job well done) and at other times alienating, especially where analgesic or anaesthetic pain relief made the woman feel she was not a participant in the birth. In Ireland, some 20 years later, Christina (see Box 8.1) describes the trauma of her birth

---

Box 8.1 Christina's story

All I remember is the fear, being left alone in bed. At ten o'clock, it was shaves and enemas. The following morning I woke up as they were wheeling me down to the labour ward. They wouldn't let me out of bed.

Then they had to catheterize me. That was the kind of communication there was in there. The nurse said, 'I'll run the taps'. I didn't know that was supposed to give you an urge to go to the toilet. I thought, what's she running the taps for? I started wondering if I was mad . . .

Why was I induced? I was two days over. I didn't have much choice about it. I was taken in on a Wednesday. At five o'clock [in the morning], they examined me and put up the drip. There was no consultation. Everyone was on a drip. You weren't asked. They broke my waters at six. It was horrendous . . . The doctor told me to fuck off and stop screaming.

I asked the sister would she ring my husband, and she said she would, but she didn't. Things like that, the loneliness . . . I felt very betrayed. The minute I stepped inside . . . You're told you will be given your own nurse but the nurse was a total stranger. And if her shift came to an end, another nurse came along, another total stranger . . .

They wouldn't let me out of bed. They would let my sister, who was a nurse, in to see me, but not my husband. The loneliness, the fear, the tiredness, that's all I remember. The stupidity of it. I was freezing cold after she was born. Nobody took a blind bit of notice.

They must have taken away half my insides. The humiliation, the tiredness, the pain . . . There was just no way I was going back to the Iveagh. It was so managed and contrived.

Source: O'Connor (1995: 20–1).

---

experience. This kind of hospital birth experience has led to growing criticism of the medical management of childbirth and to the consumer revolt in maternity services (Garcia *et al.* 1990). The pain and suffering of childbirth are described as the effects of a medicalized approach that de-humanizes and humiliates women.

How women experience their bodies is culturally mediated and bodies are constituted by discourses but are at the same time **corporeal**. In Hall's (1997a: 6) terms discourse refers to 'a cluster (or formation) or ideas, images, and practices which provide ways of talking about forms of knowledge and conduct associated with a particular topic, social activity or institutional site in society'. Pregnancy and childbirth are not therefore pre-symbolic (or 'natural'), outside language or culture, but are embodied practices (Davis 1997) occurring within specific historical, cultural and institutional settings, as discussed in preceding chapters.

The politics of representation

My focus here is on *visual representation,* the visual images of pregnancy and birth. By examining these images we can learn how the views of women, midwives, doctors and others are socially shaped and how such images create meaning, constructing experiences of pregnancy and childbirth. Different ways of thinking about 'the body' and representation influence how bodies are seen and how we may interpret images of bodies. Hall (1997a) refers to three general approaches to representation:

1 reflective: the idea that representation reflects objects or nature;
2 intentional: the idea that meaning is what the speaker or author intended;
3 constructivist: the idea that we produce meaning using symbols and signs.

Semiotics and Foucauldian discourse theory are examples of constructivist approaches. The common-sense view is often that a picture tells us, in a straightforward way, facts about a body. The ontological status of the body is not questioned, simply taken as a naturalized given. However, from a constructivist point of view, seeing these images as embedded in cultural practices means that the making of pictures, photographs and use of other visual technologies both produces meaning and constitutes women's pregnant bodies in specific ways. These *representational practices* do not simply tell us about a pre-existing body. There is no simple direct relationship between the signifier (picture) and what is signified (body).

So how are women's pregnant bodies discursively produced, or represented, using visual images in art, photography and medicine? These images do not of themselves have a fixed meaning but may be seen as part of a system of meaning and representation which is produced and consumed in diverse ways. Meanings are constantly being exchanged and interpreted – they are unstable and shifting. The *politics of representation* refers to the ways in which meanings are contested, how power intervenes, appearing to fix meaning and the struggles over other definitions and interpretations (King 1992; Hall 1997b).

In order to study culture the focus of study is 'the actual concrete forms which meaning assumes, in the concrete practices of signifying, "reading" and interpretation: and these require analysis of the actual signs, symbols, figures, images, narratives, words and sounds – the material forms – in which symbolic meaning is circulated' (Hall 1997a: 9). Visual images play an important part in constructing meaning in contemporary culture, particularly within a phallocentric or patriarchal culture (Assiter 1996; Betterton 1996). The importance of visualization as integral to medical practice demonstrates this (Martin 1990; Harrison and Aranda 1997) and is illustrated by Petchesky (1987) and stressed by Farquhar (1996). So let us consider the use of technologies of representation and how diagnostic imaging has visualized women's bodies.

Visualizing the female body – images of pregnant bodies

Historically, modern art has reflected and reproduced cultural ideals of the human figure. In his discussion of body images Mirzoeff (1995) analyses how the idealized body was both racist and fascist, perpetrating white superiority and racist science. In western art attempts were made to overcome the weakness of the physical body, to find a perfect method to represent the body and to make the imperfect body whole. In the nineteenth century, representations of women were idealized in images of the Madonna though 'the boundaries between the Madonna, the domestic woman and the fallen woman were sufficiently fluid that these categories became confused and overlapped' (Mirzoeff 1995: 98).

The work of French male artists such as Ingres are understood by Mirzoeff as an expression of male fantasy and (hetero)sexual desire. The male artists controlled female sexuality through their paintings. In their phantasmic paintings of the Oriental harim, the artists created the space to project their own European sexual repressions. The 'otherness' of women in Ingres' work was, according to Mirzoeff, 'inevitable' and the exoticism of the Oriental woman accentuated this 'otherness'. Mirzoeff says that female sexuality was deeply feared by Ingres and other artists such as Picasso and that their work exhibits an ambivalence towards the pleasures and fears of women's bodies.

Interestingly, the work of the woman photographic artist Julia Cameron is considered both similar and different from other images of the Madonna. While repeating the theme of the Madonna icon, Mirzoeff suggests that the meaning of these photographs is altered because they were taken by a woman. According to his analysis, though Cameron's intention may have been to repeat the earlier artistic work, she destabilizes its meaning, re-presenting the images of the Madonna as attraction between women.

Betterton (1996: 25) explains that artistic identity was contingent on the 'mastery' of the male artist over the female model: 'Mastery of the female nude was central to the construction of artistic identity in the nineteenth century and the site of a specifically gendered relationship'. The idealized figure in art was therefore seen through 'the male gaze' and effectively subjugated feminine subjectivity and excluded women as artists. The Madonna figure in art represents the idealized feminine form:

> the symbol of the 'virginal maternal', the impossible duality of an inviolable and fertile body which is at the heart of Christian ideals of womanhood. In representations of the Virgin Mary, the female body appears as a sealed vessel. As Lynda Nead has argued, one of the principal functions of the female nude in western art has been the containment and regulation of the female sexual body.
> (Betterton 1996: 33)

The implications of this analysis for understanding the effects of contemporary images in popular magazines such as *Pregnancy*, *Pregnancy Plus* and *Mother & Baby* written for pregnant women are important. These magazines also frequently present the pregnant woman as a sealed vessel, and often re-present a Madonna image. The picture, frequently taken from a lateral view, shows the pregnant woman standing or sitting erect, her hand resting on her abdomen symbolizing care and concern for her baby. The woman's face is usually gazing down towards her belly expectantly or turned towards the camera. A look of contentment, satisfaction and fulfilment suggests that in pregnancy the woman becomes complete,

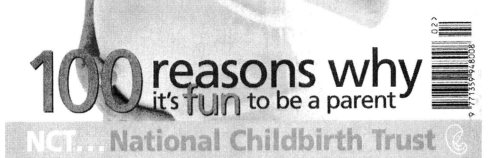

Figure 8.1 Front cover of a modern pregnancy magazine
Source: Reproduced by kind permission of NCT publishing.

her hetereosexual desire satisfied and her feminine identity fully formed (see Figure 8.1). The effects of this are to encourage women to feel and behave in certain ways. They are encouraged to see pregnancy as 'natural' and as the approved outcome of heterosex. Through these images of pregnancy the woman is defined as a 'real woman', and expected to find motherhood a rewarding and enjoyable experience. Woodward (1997) has pointed out that there are new kinds of representations of motherhood which show women as both mothers and workers, and which imply new kinds of family forms. These newer figures of motherhood also construct women's lives and bodies suggesting that pregnancy and motherhood may be combined with work. Woodward also drew my attention to images of pregnant women at work, though these are not widespread.

Women as artists

Betterton (1996) discusses how the position of women artists is a contradictory one, how being an artist and being a woman were, and to an extent still are, in conflict. At the centre of her discussion is an analysis of the politics of representation and a politicization of aesthetic values. Through the practices of painting and representation the male artist created women as objects through the male gaze. Both the technique of painting (the method of representation) and the symbolic significance of the blank canvas were brought under the control of the painter and perpetuated the relationship between model and artist. The male artist observed and looked, while the female model was looked upon and created as an object on the canvas. Women artists painting nudes therefore confront directly 'inscription of the gender difference on the body' (Betterton 1996: 25).

Following Betterton's analysis, becoming a female artist is transgressive and destabilizes the artistic norms that have prevailed throughout history:

> Those images by women which combine self-portraiture with the nude articulate the problem of representing this psychic split between feminine and artistic subjectivity. [But] A self-portrait, like the act of writing a journal, or a letter, constructs the self as other, making available to others a particular representation of the subject which the author has selected. The autobiographical is thus not the unmediated expression of inner being, but the production of a fictive self which functions as a form of self 're-presentation'.
>
> (Betterton 1996: 26)

For a woman this is more problematic than for a man because, according to Betterton, she confronts the conflict between the public and private selves (see also Borzello 1998).

The pregnant nude

In her discussion of the work of twentieth-century German female artist Paula Modersohn-Becker, Betterton (1996) examines the self-portrait of the artist imagining herself pregnant. In Germany becoming a mother previously meant the loss of artistic identity, as mothers could not become artists. Betterton suggests that Becker uses pregnancy as a metaphor, a fantasy, by representing herself as pregnant, as 'other'. By combining a nude self-portrait with an imaginary pregnancy Becker symbolizes the lost identity of maternity and 'disavows it'. For Betterton, the painting enables the artist to transcend the loss of identity associated with actual motherhood, to represent a condition that is between the identity of artist and mother.

In another detailed discussion of Paula Modersohn-Becker's work and her attitudes towards pregnancy and childbirth Hansch (1997) suggests that the artist saw no contradiction between artistic and maternal identity. In contrast she argues that it is pregnancy and childbirth which become the carriers of individuality and that this self-portrait was the utmost expression of individuality. Borzello (1998: 144) suggests that this is the 'archetypal pregnancy pose' (see Figure 8.2).

The pregnant nude may be seen as a paradox, a contradiction in terms. While 'virgin mothers' represent a sealed vessel, earthly mothers lose their identity, or it is split:

> But if, as Nead suggests, the function of the nude is to make 'safe' the permeable borderline between nature and culture, the maternal body potentially disrupts that boundary. For the maternal body points to the impossibility of closure, to a liminal state where the boundaries of the body are fluid. In the act of giving birth, as well as during pregnancy and breastfeeding, the body of the mother is the subject of a constant exchange with that of the child. Whereas the nude is seamless, the pregnant body signifies the state in which the boundaries of inside and outside, self and other, dissolve.
>
> (Betterton 1996: 33)

In 1992 the photograph of performing artist Demi Moore on the cover of *Vanity Fair* was controversial. As a pregnant nude of a famous, public figure, the photograph confronted the conflict between the public and private selves. It made pregnancy visible, in a public way, glamorizing and sexualizing the pregnant body. Indeed the visibility of pregnant bodies is usually strictly controlled. Images of pregnant bodies are not widely and readily available except in the limited contexts of the hospital, mother and baby books or magazines. In these contexts motherhood is medicalized and normalized and the idea of a pregnant woman as a sexualized subject remains ambivalent and controversial in the public imagination (Walton 1994).

Fragmenting subjectivity

Betterton's remarks above about the instability of the boundaries of the pregnant body echo the words of Iris Young (1984). She also says that pregnancy 'dissolves' and fragments unitary notions of subjectivity. She describes fragmentation as central to the experience of being pregnant. The pregnant woman 'experiences her body as herself and not herself. Its inner movements belong to another being, yet they are not other, because

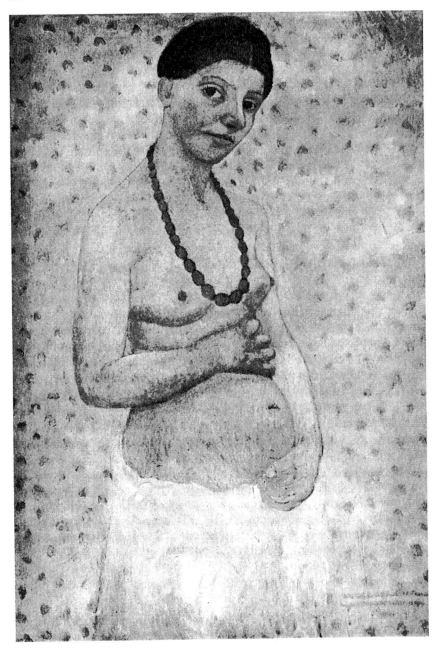

Figure 8.2 Paula Modersohn-Becker, *Self Portrait on Her Sixth Wedding Day*
Source: Reproduced by permission of Paula Modersohn-Becker Museum, Böttcherstrasse, Bremen.

her body boundaries shift and because her bodily self-location is focused on her trunk in addition to her head' (Young 1984: 46). The integrity of the body is undermined in pregnancy, says Young, and the pregnant woman has no firm sense of where she ends and the world begins. She struggles sometimes to maintain previous bodily habits – 'habits which retain the old sense of [her] boundaries' (1984: 49), to move where previously she could move with ease. In pregnancy the woman is newly aware of her body. Young argues for this new awareness as a positive circumstance which is 'aesthetically interesting' to the woman. Rather than seeing her body as an alienated object which gets in the way, her 'relation to her body can be an innocent narcissism' (1984: 53), observed by her and mobilized in her actions with intention and agency. For Young, the pregnant subject is an active one, not simply expectant and waiting, though medical discourse and practice usually defines the pregnant body as an object to be acted *upon*.

Ways of seeing – diagnostic imaging

In conventional accounts of science in general and medical science in particular, claims are made for scientific knowledge to be separate from culture. As already indicated in Chapter 2 such claims have been challenged. In her book *The Woman in the Body* Martin (1993) explores the idea of science as a cultural system and examines the medical metaphors of women's bodies. She shows how ideas of women's bodies changed over time but that metaphors were important in how medicine developed and also how women viewed their own bodies.

Menstruation and menopause were understood as based on metaphors of the body as a small business with an intake-outgo system, a factory in industrial capitalist society, and subsequently as an information-transmitting system organized hierarchically. From the nineteenth century menstruation and menopause were pathologized, seen as failed production and/or a breakdown in organization and hierarchy respectively. In both cases negative terms were used to describe these bodily processes such as degeneration, decay and failure. Childbirth was understood, since the seventeenth and eighteenth century, in terms of the body as machine, the uterus seen as a machine to push the baby out. In those days, Martin (1993) suggests, the use of forceps and the role of the doctor was similar to that of a mechanic and to an extent this view of the doctor as technical expert has persisted, though in modified form. Certainly the criticisms of Oakley (1986) and others were that women in childbirth became extensions to the machines and paraphernalia of medical technologies (see Figure 8.3).

Martin (1993: 63) analyses the idea of the labouring woman as a labourer/worker and considers the extent to which this is compatible with the metaphor of body as machine. She concludes that 'medical imagery juxtaposes two pictures: the uterus as a machine that produces the baby and the woman as a labourer who produces the baby. Perhaps at times the two come together as the woman-labourer whose uterus-machine produces the baby'.

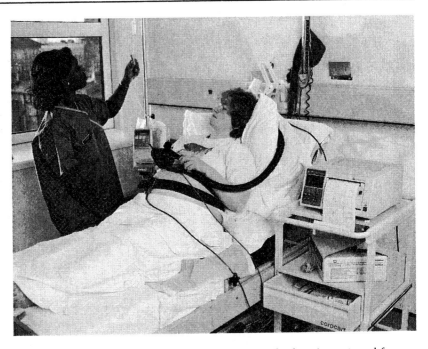

Figure 8.3 The image of a woman attached to medical equipment used for
pain relief and to monitor labour
Source: Reproduced by permission of MIDIRS (Midwives Information and Resource Service).

These ideas are now easily recognizable as integral to the biomedical
model of pregnancy and childbirth which I discussed in Chapter 2. This
model constitutes the woman's body as object, managed and acted upon
by the doctor. This process of objectification, as we saw, is strongly criticized
by many feminists writing about women's maternity and health care.

Visualizing the foetus

Surveillance of women during pregnancy and childbirth was considered
by Oakley (1986) to be a primary objective for modern maternity care. As
she discusses, the development of ultrasound technology in the 1950s
signalled an extension of medical surveillance to the foetus. Intrauterine
visualization of the foetus she says facilitated access to it in a way that
was unprecedented. It seemed that the doctor no longer needed to direct
questions to the pregnant woman about the foetus, but observed for
himself the foetus in the womb. In a sense the mother was obliterated
(Harrison and Aranda 1997) and women were reconfigured 'as objects of
mechanical surveillance rather than recipients of antenatal care' (Oakley
1986: 159).

   As Bordo (1995) and Petchesky (1987) argue, this process of visualization assisted in the creation of the foetus as a subject, especially in abortion debates and legal discourse. As a person, the mother is absent from

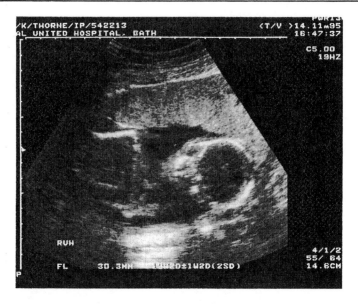

Figure 8.4 An ultrasound scan of foetus *in utero*
Source: Reproduced by permission of John and Karen Thorne.

the picture and becomes an object, the incubator and container for the
foetus. Her subjectivity and personhood is erased (see also Shildrick 1997)
and her womb is seen as a window on the foetus or 'a frame which is
meaningful only in relation to the figure it delimits' (Adams 1994: 156).
Bordo, quoting Harrison puts it like this:

> The foetus could not be taken seriously as long as he remained a
> medical recluse in an opaque womb; and it was not until the last half
> of this century that the prying eye of the ultrasonogram rendered the
> once opaque womb transparent, stripping the veil of mystery from
> the dark inner sanctum, and letting the light of scientific observation
> fall on the shy and secretive foetus.
>
> (Bordo 1995: 85)

The personhood of the foetus is represented in opposition to that of the
mother who provides the maternal space. Even in so-called 'alternative'
approaches to childbirth such as the Leboyer method discussed by Adams,
the mother is 'enemy' and birth is a struggle to break free (Adams 1994).
The obstetrician intervenes to 'rescue' the child (see Figure 8.4).

Observation as scientific method

The concept of surveillance has been important for understanding the
ways in which bodies have been disciplined and regulated. According to
Foucault (1979, 1985, 1990) and others such as Turner (1992) 'the body
represents a regulatory problem in the development of human civilisa-
tion' (Turner, 1992: 13). Observation has been the method of surveillance

and (as we saw in Chapter 2) the growth of large-scale institutions such as the hospital facilitated this. Foucault's (1973) account of *The Birth of the Clinic* and 'panopticanism' highlighted the importance attached to visualization. The 'clinical gaze' is primarily directed towards the twin purposes of regulation and discipline. As Martin reminds us, 'in Western thought the illumination that vision gives has been associated with the highest faculty of mental reasoning' and 'vision has been a primary route to scientific knowledge' (Martin 1990: 69). Observation as a method was accorded high status in the sciences through the use of the microscope (Harrison 1995). Harrison and Aranda (1997), in their discussion of photography and medicine, consider how the development of clinical practice was closely linked to skills of observation and new technologies of photography.

The medical photograph, they tell us, was primarily concerned with observing and recording the 'extraordinary', the 'abnormal'. Initially such photographs were used to observe the exterior of the body, its surface characteristics and shape, to mark 'visible difference'. 'Pathology was seeable' and even in the context of psychiatric photography outward appearance was thought to relate to inner pathology. Medical photographs of women emphasized the power of the male observer and the links between the male gaze and the clinical gaze. Drawing on earlier research Harrison and Aranda (1997) remark on the prevalence of photographs of Victorian mad*women*. Women were more likely to be diagnosed as abnormal.

The development of new technologies such as X-rays, ultrasonography and more recently fibreoptic endoscopy and tomography provided the chance to visualize the inside of the body. But these new ways of seeing do not simply reveal what is inside, rather, as Harrison and Aranda (1997) say, what is seen had to be learnt, a new 'visual literacy' developed. The content of images had to be interpreted and such interpretations are historically located and socially produced (Petechsky 1987). These technologies produced images of pregnancy that created a different relationship between obstetricians and their newly-constituted patient – the foetus. Relationships with mothers were also transformed, as the mother was erased, becoming the background to the foetal subject, 'framed' in the womb (see Figure 8.4). Through the processes of visualization and representation, power was exercised with both positive and negative effects. Power in the Foucauldian sense is both productive and disciplinary, constituting both the subjects and objects of knowledge (Foucault 1973; Turner 1992; Harrison and Aranda 1997).

Leaking bodies – the female gaze and feminine subjectivity

So far I have argued that images of women were idealized in the paintings of the Madonna. The virginal mother represented a sealed vessel and I have suggested that some images of earthly mothers appear also to represent the pregnant body as a sealed vessel, an object to be looked upon. The idealized maternal subject has also been seen as complete and fulfilled in pregnancy. However, the nude pregnant body is at the same time contradictory because it points to the impossibility of closure in the female body

(Betterton 1996) and the splitting of subjectivity. Though a nude is seam-less, during pregnancy and childbirth the boundaries between self and other, inside and outside become blurred. Some feminist writings on the female body see this blurring of boundaries as representing a fundamental challenge to ideas about the modern subject, as we shall see.

A second way in which pregnant women are represented is as 'incubators' where only the foetus in the womb is seen and the foetus is constituted as a subject separate from the mother. The mother in these cases is obliter-ated, absent or erased from view. Feminist concerns to reconstitute women as subjects, as part of a modernist project of emancipation, highlight the effects of such a view (Petchesky 1987). For them the (bodily) presence of the woman in the picture is important for her political recognition. Yet the very idea of the feminine subject may be seen as problematic (Shildrick 1997).

The feminine subject – individuality and femininity

In her work *Anorexic Bodies* MacSween argues that there is a tension between the exterior surface of the feminine body and the interior, in ways which mean that 'bodily closure is [exclusively] a masculine possibility' (1993: 173) (see also Bordo 1995). Although women may strive for bodily integ-rity whereby the external surface of the body appears as a closed and flaw-less boundary, this is ultimately not achievable. Through beauty regimes such as skin care the woman seeks to create a boundary between the interior of her body and the exterior for 'the perfected skin offers no way in, its boundaries are firm and clear – they do not yield' (MacSween 1993: 178).

According to MacSween's analysis, in bourgeous culture, 'the individual' is a masculine subject with a masculine body, separate from the environ-ment but able to act upon it. In contrast the feminine body is constructed as the environment for the masculine self, the space which men fill, an object where the physicality or corporeality of the body is all a woman is. The womb symbolizes this space (Adams 1994; Grosz 1995; Shildrick 1997). There is therefore a contradiction between individuality and femininity in patriarchal culture and:

> For women such psychosomatic harmony does not exist, the dominant body-concept co-exists for women with the 'sub-text' of femininity. In this women's selves, as well as their bodies, are objects in the masculine environment, and their 'boundaries' are fluid and penetrable rather than self-contained and invasive.
>
> (MacSween 1993: 54)

Anorexia seems to offer some women a way of resolving this conflict between individuality and femininity and by not taking in food (symbolic-ally) the woman closes herself off from the environment. She attempts to create a body surface that is impenetrable, that is 'absolute' and a body shape that is lean and more masculine than feminine. This view of anor-exia explains why a denial of feminine openness and fluidity offers the anorexic woman the promise of selfhood. By disciplining and controlling her appetite, which threatens to destroy her self, the woman intends to create her self as separate, clean, integrated and whole. For anorexic women the importance of body shape is linked to this claim to selfhood. The desire for thinness is not simply a naive response to the pressures of the beauty industry, but an understandable response to dominant phallocentric cultural values and aspirations to become an autonomous individual.

Bodily boundaries

As part of a modernist project, the dilemma for women is how to become full political subjects in an economy where a woman's body does not, and cannot attain the masculine possibility of being a closed, separate and bounded system (Shildrick 1997). Constituted instead as objects to be looked upon, women's subjectivity is constantly undermined. Pregnancy, as Young (1984, 1990) suggests, represents a paradigmatic case of split subjectivity. The connections of one to another radically undermine the notion of the autonomous individual. It is for this reason that Betterton (1996) suggests the Benneton advertisement which showed the new-born baby apparently still attached to its mother was controversial (see Figure 8.5). Such an image subverted the accepted view that individuals and bodies are separate from each other. Betterton says the image represented Kristeva's (1982) idea of the horrific by collapsing the border between inside and outside, self and other, unsettling bodily boundaries and threatening identity.

Similarly, Gallop explains that the image of a woman giving birth on the cover of her book *Thinking Through the Body* (1988) is intentionally ambiguous and her aim is to disrupt convention. She says:

> I chose a photograph that shows the head in the midst of the body . . . I wanted to put an image of the body on the front cover that was not neatly placed, that might still have the power to disturb. It was suggested that the nurse be cropped out to make the photo easier to read. I like the entanglement, the difficulty in sorting out one body from another.
>
> (Gallop 1988: 8)

For Gallop, opposition between philosophers and mothers, thinkers and bodies exemplifies the mind-body split. The head, in the middle of the body, she argues, is a case for relocating thinking – to see it as *embodied*, and as something women do. Yet, she tells us some people find such a picture 'gross'.

Images of women giving birth are disruptive and challenging because they show the interdependence of one body on another and represent the 'horror' of a leaky body (Kristeva cited in Betterton 1996). Cultural studies of menstruation such as Martin's (1990) have highlighted the negative meanings attached to it by women, men and the medical profession. Rather than a celebration of the female body, both menstruation and menopause are constituted as failures or degenerative processes. The terms and metaphors used to describe the menstrual cycle, Martin shows, imply that 'leaky bodies' are problematic. This horror of 'leakiness' is also evident in cultural attitudes towards incontinence and other uncontrolled loss of bodily fluid (Shildrick 1997).

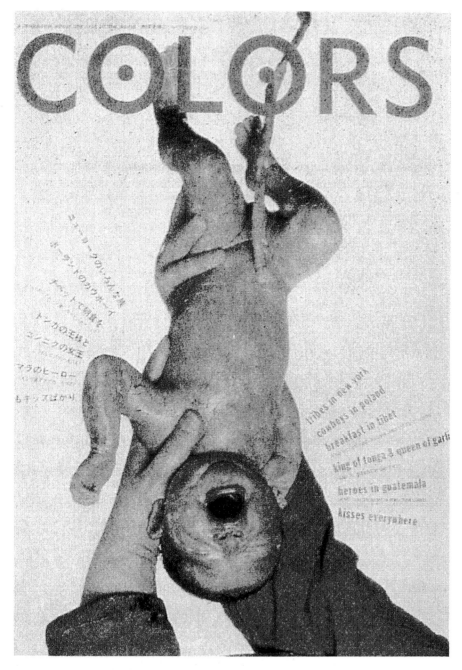

Figure 8.5   Benetton 'Baby' advertisement, 1991
Source: Reproduced by permission of Benetton, photograph by Oliviero Toscani.

Feminist practice

What feminist artists, photographers and critical theorists suggest are alternative ways of seeing women's bodies. The well-known photographer Jo
Spence used photography as a form of *Cultural Sniping* (1995) a way of
'putting [her] self in the picture' (Spence 1986) and of developing 'a
female gaze'. As King (1992) explains the politics of representation are a
politics of meaning, of how signs are used to signify what it means to be
a woman. Visual ideologies construct available kinds of images of pregnant bodies. 'The consumption of visual images is dangerously asym-
metrical. Most images are made by men for men' (King 1992: 133). Spence
and other feminist artists seek to use other signs to represent leakiness,
softness, fatness, disease and other aspects of female bodies. Such work
attempts to reframe how we think, see and know our bodies and empower
women as viewers of bodies, as subjects rather than objects. As Petchesky
(1987: 79) argues the challenge is to create a new image of the pregnant
woman 'not as an abstraction, but within her total framework of relationships, economic and health needs and desires'.

This project is not straightforward and there is no agreement about
what form it might take or what constitutes 'a female gaze'. Indeed the
very notion of 'a female gaze' presupposes that there is a direct relationship between the bodily experience of having a female body and representing 'femininity'. If, as discussed already, the connections between sex
and gender are loosened then it is not simply the case that a female artist
reveals her femininity in her work. Rather, femininity itself may be seen
as a product of phallocentric culture – a system of masculinist signs and
values. Within psychoanalytic theory seeing one's image in the mirror has
been seen as important for developing a sense of oneself, and for identity
formation. However, feminists have been critical of these ideas arguing
that the prioritizing of visual images within the symbolic order is a
masculinist construct. Irigaray's work (see Chapter 6) has contributed to
debate about whether 'a female gaze' reproduces an essentialist view of
the feminine subject (Fuss 1989; Assiter 1996; Betterton 1996). She argues
for a different symbolic order, for a system of signs which enables women
to speak as women, rather than to be confined by the representations and
symbols of a system that denies them full citizenship or subjecthood
(Irigaray 1985a, 1985b; Whitford 1991; Grosz 1995; Assiter 1996). However, this is not necessarily to suggest that femininity or the bodily experiences of being a woman mean the same thing to everyone or are fixed.
Rather, the work of feminist artists and photographers suggests that the
way meanings are visually coded may be contested in diverse ways.

By seeing images of pregnancy and childbirth as having social and
political significance it becomes important to deconstruct them, to examine how power relations produce certain views of women and their pregnant bodies. The possibility then of alternatives begins to come into view.
For example, recognizing the political significance of visual images, the
Spinal Injuries Association and Righting the Picture, a visual project supported by the National Childbirth Trust, present images of disabled men
and women as parents. The picture of a disabled pregnant woman shown
in Figure 8.6 challenges directly the assumptions that disability always

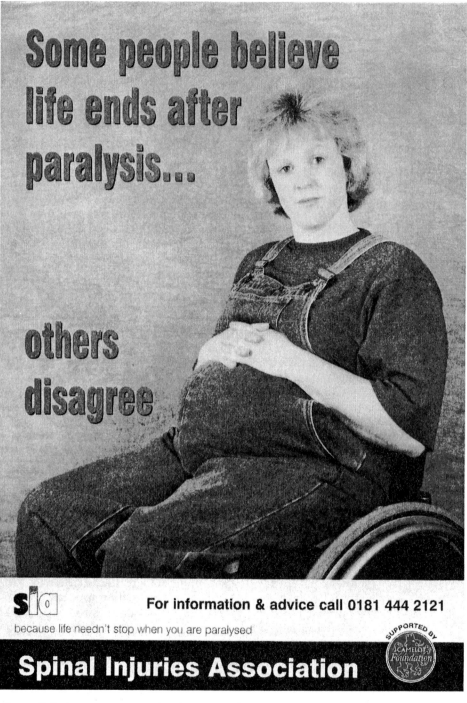

Figure 8.6 A poster campaign by the Spinal Injuries Association to promote positive images of disability and parenthood
Source: Reproduced by kind permission of the Spinal Injuries Association/Jim Kelly.

precludes pregnancy or childbirth. Other images of intimacy, desire and erotic bodies (Buurman 1997) signal that disabled bodies may participate in sexual activity and be seen as both attractive and desirable (see Chapter 6).

Conclusions

In this chapter I have sought to outline the debates about how bodies are theorized. While my earlier discussion of sexual identities explored in more detail the connections between sex, gender and sexuality, the focus of this chapter has been the ways in which representational practices construct meanings of pregnancy, childbirth and the maternal subject.

Historically, the dominant image in figurative art has been the Madonna, the virgin mother represented as an idealized sealed vessel, an object to be looked upon. In medical practice the visualization of women's bodies has emphasized the pathological and the abnormal. More recently, with the development of new technologies, views of the inside of the womb have had the effect of erasing the woman. Instead the woman as incubator became the dominant image and the foetus was constituted as a subject separate from its mother.

Pregnancy and childbirth may be seen as the paradigmatic case of a split subjectivity where the notion of a modern, humanist subject is radically undermined. In pregnancy the boundaries between inside and outside may be seen as blurred – the beginning and end of one body is unclear, as exemplified in images of childbirth and Young's (1984, 1990) phenomenological account of pregnancy. This connection of the maternal subject to an 'other' is what some feminists argue points to the need to rethink the boundaries of the body. Maternity is associated with a loss of a unitary identity – instead these bodily experiences contribute to a sense of fragmentation.

At the same time this splitting and fragmentation, this 'leakiness' can be seen as representing the postmodern condition (Shildrick 1997). This is a condition where the boundaries between bodies, between selves and others, human and machine become increasingly unclear. However a view of the human condition which loses sight of embodied practices such as pregnancy and giving birth arguably loses sight of what it is to be human. For while these visual images and other representational practices configure 'women' or 'mothers' in certain ways, giving meaning to being a woman or being a mother, pregnant bodies are also corporeal. While we have access to these bodily experiences through representational practices this is not the sum total of what we are. As corporeal or material bodies there are physical limits to what we do and how we live but these are always culturally mediated. There is a tension between the symbolic and the material that is embodied in these experiences. There is therefore nothing 'natural' about being pregnant or giving birth that is outside culture. The experiences of women who become pregnant and give birth may only be understood within the context of a social world and it is for this reason that we need to be able to analyse those experiences from a sociological perspective.

The implications of the politics of representation are important for health care practitioners because they assist in understanding how different forms of knowledge are constructed. Medical practice is traditionally underpinned by a reliance on scientific knowledge and, as already suggested, other health care practitioners have also sought to develop a more 'scientific' approach. However, power relations are constituted through the production of knowledge, and discourse theory highlights the connections between knowledge and power. Women's experiences of pregnancy and childbirth are embodied practices whereby discourses, institutions and bodies intersect. The identities of 'mother' and 'woman' are discursively produced through the cultural processes of signification and representation. It follows therefore that both health care practitioners and women are engaged in a politics of representation, exchanging meanings and understandings. Rather than constantly reproducing a male or clinical gaze, health care practitioners need to develop a critical analysis of these processes and to assist in democratizing the gaze (King 1992). This means creating the space for different points of view and negotiating the form and meaning of 'health care' during pregnancy and childbirth.

Summary

- In social theory increasingly bodies are seen as central to social action. The biological and the social are seen as interlinked.

- For many years feminist writers have highlighted the ways in which women's bodies have been oppressed and abused. The meanings attached to women's bodies and bodily functions such as menstruation and menopause have been particularly negative.

- Women's experiences of their bodies and of reproduction have been socially constructed through cultural processes of signification and representation.

- These processes of signification and representation include both artistic and scientific practices. Traditionally both artists and scientists have been men and have constructed images of women's bodies as objects of heterosexual desire to be gazed upon, regulated and controlled.

- Techniques of painting, photography and diagnostic imaging have incorporated specific 'ways of seeing' women and mothers. Pregnancy has been represented as a state of fulfilment and contentment for women.

- In contrast, women artists, photographers and writers have represented pregnancy and childbirth in alternative ways. Maternal subjectivity has been seen as problematic and women's 'leaky bodies' as representative of 'the postmodern condition'.

- The pregnant woman potentially disrupts (patriarchal) ideologies of autonomy and individualism because pregnancy connects one body to another and thereby subverts the notion of a unitary identity.

- By recognizing the links between knowledge, power, bodies and identity, the effects of categorizing women, or mothers, and treating them as an homogenous and unified group begin to come into view.
- The health care professional, by developing an understanding of different ways of seeing and knowing the world, may negotiate with pregnant women the meaning and forms of 'maternity care'.

Discussion points

- To what extent do doctors and midwives naturalize and universalize bodies?
- Why is a binary divide between nature and culture unsatisfactory?
- How are pregnancy and childbirth socially constructed?
- How are pregnancy and childbirth represented in popular magazines?
- In what sense is the notion of a maternal subject a problem?
- Why is embodiment important in thinking about bodies?

Further reading

Betterton, R. (1996) *An Intimate Distance: Women, Artists and the Body*. London: Routledge.

Bonner, F., Goodman, L., Allen, R., Janes, L. and King, C. (eds) (1992) *Imagining Women: Cultural Representations and Gender*. Cambridge: Polity Press.

Davis, K. (ed.) (1997) *Embodied Practices: Feminist Perspectives on the Body*. London: Sage.

Hall, S. (ed.) (1997) *Representation: Cultural Representations and Signifying Practices*. Buckingham: Open University Press.

Petchesky, R. (1987) Foetal images: the power of visual culture in the politics of reproduction, in M. Stanworth (ed.) *Reproductive Technologies: Gender, Motherhood and Medicine*. Oxford: Blackwell.

Shildrick, M. (1997) *Leaky Bodies and Boundaries: Feminism, Postmodernism and (Bio)ethics*. London: Routledge.

NINE

CHANGING CHILDBIRTH, CHANGING THE FUTURE?

Introduction
Democracy in the NHS
Revaluing care
Acknowledging difference
Re-visioning the future
Summary

Introduction

The intention of this book has been to assist midwives, nurses and other health care professionals to develop a sociological perspective on pregnancy and childbirth. I began by suggesting that in the past there has been a separation between the biological and social sciences and this may be seen as linked to broad historical processes. More recently in social theory the links between the biological and the social aspects of human existence have been seen as important. Although previously social theorists took for granted the biological base of social action and focused on social structures and processes, this was heavily criticized, particularly by feminists. Feminists were critical of these assumptions because biology was seen as an explanation of gender inequalities and this was discredited. Much feminist writing has been around reproduction since pregnancy and childbirth are important aspects of many, though not all, women's lives. Even the lives of women who do not become pregnant or give birth have been shaped by attitudes towards sex, sexuality, reproduction and motherhood (see Chapters 5, 6 and 7).

Feminists have argued that social relations between men and women have been shaped by dominant patriarchal values that underpinned traditional forms of 'the family' and also affected women's working lives (see Chapters 2 and 4). Patriarchy was characterized as valuing certain kinds of knowledge through which power has been exercised over women's lives and women's bodies. Scientific knowledge, despite its claim to impartiality, objectivity and universalism, was seen as privileging white, heterosexual men. This was exemplified by the historical rise of obstetrics as a branch of medicine that increasingly marginalized the knowledge and experience of traditional midwives (see Chapter 2).

Historically, midwives and the medical profession have been seen as engaged in a struggle over professional territory. This struggle, which dates back to the nineteenth century, was linked to the development of modern health care systems and the growth of professional knowledge. In order to ensure that midwives had a role in the emerging maternity services, according to some, compromises were made about the scope of their responsibilities (Witz 1992). Although legally responsible for her own practice and professionally accountable to the regulatory bodies set up at that time, the midwife was expected to refer pregnant women to the doctor under certain circumstances. This legal framework has been sustained, though modified by subsequent Acts (see Chapter 2). The position of midwives today has therefore been structured by gender relations.

Since the early 1990s there have been changes in the organization of midwifery and nurse education (see Chapter 3). These changes have occurred alongside a growing concern among midwives to develop a stronger knowledge base. The proliferation of nursing and midwifery textbooks is evidence of this (for example: Robinson and Vaughan 1993; Bryar 1995; Perry 1997). In developing this knowledge, and in the light of the relocation of health care education within higher education, midwives and nurses increasingly draw on the theories and concepts of the social sciences (Hunt and Symonds 1995; Ackers and Abbott 1996; Payne and Walker 1996; Symonds and Hunt 1996; Bephage 1997). Curriculum changes have led to the inclusion of a range of additional topics and materials in the education programme. An understanding of both social and feminist theory is seen as useful for health care practitioners (Walton 1994; Davies 1995; Wilton 1997; Porter 1998; Miers, forthcoming). In this final chapter I hope to draw together the central themes of this book and to show how feminist sociological perspectives on pregnancy and childbirth may be useful for health care practice.

Democracy in the NHS

One central theme throughout this book has been the connections between knowledge and power. The discussion of professional power pointed to the ability of doctors, midwives and other health care professionals to exercise control over the lives of those seeking maternity services. The shape and form of health services has in the past been seen as serving the interests of powerful professionals rather than patients or service users. As Doyal (1998: 3) points out:

> Though the NHS represented a major step forward in the organisation and financing of healthcare it was never a model for democratic planning. Few mechanisms of accountability or participation were built into the system with the result that the majority of users (and most workers) have had little opportunity to influence its operation.

Doyal suggests however that things are changing as a result of the reorganization of the NHS in the 1980s and the development of the managed market with purchaser and provider roles (see also Ackers and Abbott

1996). In the area of maternity services long-standing criticisms made about the quality and kind of services available were seen as the background to *Changing Childbirth* (Department of Health 1993). Both consumer groups and midwives successfully argued for change. I discussed these proposals for change to a 'woman-centred' service and the idea that women's own knowledge and experience of their bodies, their needs and wishes, might be accorded greater significance (Chapter 2).

While there is evidence of some improvements, and the recognition of consumer demands for a better service was welcomed, the extent to which changes have benefited women is contested. Women continue to be disadvantaged in the NHS as both workers and as service users and there is continuing evidence that some women still do not receive adequate or appropriate treatments in areas such as family planning, abortion services, sexual health and fertility treatments (Doyal 1998; Thomas 1998). Those groups most likely to have their needs unmet are lesbian women, black and ethnic minority women and disabled women (Asch and Fine 1997; Wilton 1997, 1998; Douglas 1998). Starkey (1998) says that although the 1993 report *Changing Childbirth* recognized the importance of link and advocacy workers for non-English speaking women needing maternity care, few schemes have been set up. Where schemes, such as the one she describes in Bristol (which was established earlier, in 1984), have been successful, Starkey says that the new 'contract culture' in health services creates difficulties for these workers. What seems evident is that while policies have changed, the process of implementation and the extent to which health care practice has been transformed is a more complex issue. I argued that an emphasis on greater choice and control for women sometimes takes for granted a particular view of women as consumers and as autonomous subjects (see Chapter 2 and 7). However, choices are structured by unequal access to resources, especially knowledge and power. Making health care professionals accountable for their practice remains difficult and is currently under review by government.

A review of the ways in which the health care professions are regulated is in progress and there are proposals for changes in the structure and function of the regulatory bodies which are responsible for nursing and midwifery (ENB 1998a; JM Consulting Ltd 1998; UKCC 1998). For all health care practitioners, professional accountability is linked to the ability to be self-governing and midwives have fought hard to secure this right. What I hope to have shown here is that such a claim is contingent on the valuing of certain kinds of knowledge and the political struggle for a professional identity (see Chapters 2, 3 and 4). While formal education and training for professional practice has been important in establishing standards of care and guidelines for practice, other consequences flow from this. My hope is that nurses, midwives and other health care practitioners will understand and recognize what those other effects are. In particular how the alignment of professional interests with those of client groups is problematic. Inequalities persist and need to be acknowledged. Knowledge is not a neutral commodity which may be mobilized for the mutual benefit of all – rather, knowledge positions people in specific ways and there are different types and theories of knowledge as indicated throughout this book.

Revaluing care

From the discussion of midwifery work (see Chapter 4) and women as mothers (see Chapter 5) we saw that caring has not generally been defined as a skilled task. Instead, caring work has been traditionally defined as 'women's work' and consistently undervalued. Health care work and caring for children, with a focus on bodily needs and desires, has been regarded as something which women do 'naturally' and has attracted fewer rewards in terms of either social status or pay. Midwives have frequently taken for granted the view that midwifery is, and should be, 'women's work' in an effort to protect their jobs and form alliances 'with women'. The effects of this have not always been as intended for these arguments reinforce a binary gender divide. In the longer term this may discourage and prevent men from becoming either paid carers (such as nurses and midwives) or unpaid carers in the home (see Chapter 4). I supported the view that caring can be seen as a skill and that as such both mothers and midwives have a right to expect better rewards for what they do. At the same time however, the 'naturalness' of these skills needs to be called into question.

In Chapter 5 I argued that although the majority of women have the potential to become pregnant and give birth this need not necessarily imply that they have a natural ability to mother or care for children. Theories of mothering have supported traditional gender roles within 'the family' and reproduced inequalities. The suggestion that women are 'natural' carers has had the effect of excluding them from access to certain kinds of paid work and shaped social policies in ways that have not been of benefit to them. Many women care for children in conditions of poverty and material deprivation. The 'male breadwinner model' has continued to shape attitudes towards lone mothers and cohabiting mothers (Millar 1996). There is continuing evidence of the negative effects of caring, both in the home and at work, on women's health.

An increased emphasis on 'evidence-based practice' has permeated the educational and professional literature (Walsh and Crompton 1997; ENB 1998b). What needs to be considered carefully is just what counts as evidence? An understanding of both social and biological aspects of health is needed and a recognition of different methodologies to examine these different aspects. While the use of biological indicators of health has a long tradition, the value of asking women about their experiences of maternity care is less well established outside the social sciences. Increasingly though such accounts may be seen as an important way of assessing the value of 'care'. The similarities and differences between 'expert knowledge' and lay accounts of health care point to ways in which each are socially constructed. Frequently in maternity care women are constituted as both objects and subjects of knowledge. As outlined in *Changing Childbirth* (Department of Health 1993), and recognized by some practitioners, dialogue between health care professionals and those they care for is important for negotiating the most appropriate way to meet the health care needs and desires of the parturient woman. However, the conditions for such a dialogue need to be carefully understood and need not presuppose that the identity of those who participate is either fixed or unitary.

Acknowledging difference

The knowledge of who we are, and want we need, or want, is a complex issue (see Chapters 5 and 6). Sex differences have been largely taken for granted as self-evident and as underpinning gender roles. However, the biological basis of social difference has been hotly contested. Feminists have been critical of health services and health care practitioners for failing to take account of both sex and gender differences. Medical research has been criticized for failing to include women in studies; few women have been able to enter health service management and studies suggest that women are discriminated against in certain treatment areas (Doyal 1998). In the area of maternity care, where the focus is women, practices such as the routine screening of women's bodies antenatally have been criticized for failing to differentiate between women's needs, and for making assumptions about the desirability of such services. The organization and availability of fertility treatments and contraceptive services have also been criticized for inadequate care of some women (Thomas 1998). These criticisms, as well as drawing attention to areas of health care practice that might be improved, highlight the importance of acknowledging differences between women.

The discussion of women as mothers (see Chapter 5) and sexual identities (see Chapter 6) showed how the construction of 'difference' has frequently led to disadvantage and discrimination. Heterosexist ideology emphasizes sexual differences as the primary means of categorization and identification. Similarly, racist ideology categorizes people on the basis of skin colour and racial stereotyping. This biological reductionism has been heavily criticized for failing to explain the processes of discrimination and social disadvantage. Moreover, the gender divide between men and women has been seen as a binary divide that supports patriarchy. Instead I argued that we need to recognize how social differences become embodied and how 'sex' is assigned. Acknowledging difference is important to enable equal and fair treatment. Such differences, rather than being seen as tied to biology, must be seen as unstable, contested and socially produced. Identity, rather than being fixed and unitary, or a simple categorization as 'man' or 'woman', must be seen instead as fluid and changing in different social and historical contexts (Woodward 1997).

Recognizing the significance of difference means examining health care practice to see how such differences may be accommodated (Gerrish *et al.* 1996a, 1996b). For example, it cannot be assumed that all pregnant women are 'heterosexual, married and happy to be mothers' (Symonds and Hunt 1996: 119). Rather than seeing sexuality as 'a problem' for nurses and midwives its definition as 'a problem' can be seen as socially constructed. This implies that the problem is social and professional attitudes towards sexuality, and how these affect the care of, for example, lesbian women during pregnancy and childbirth. Similarly, by adopting a social model of disability, it becomes clearer that disability is not reducible to physical impairment but is socially produced. Lack of access to treatment and resources and prejudice towards women with disabilities becoming pregnant, or caring for children, marginalizes and excludes these women.

Providing additional and appropriate support for women from ethnic minority groups seeking maternity care also means acknowledging difference and responding positively.

Re-visioning the future

At the centre of this discussion about pregnancy and childbirth are women's bodies. Throughout this book I have tried to show that pregnancy and childbirth are embodied practices mediated by social and cultural processes. There is nothing natural or pre-discursive about pregnancy or childbirth because the way women see themselves, and how they experience these events is culturally and socially constructed. Dominant ideas about women as mothers (see Chapter 5) suggest that pregnancy and childbirth represent a state of fulfilment and completeness for women (see Chapter 8). Women are most frequently defined in relation to their bodies as having potential to reproduce and give birth. The normative effects of this view pervade much health care.

In the area of fertility treatment we saw that the desire for a child was considered natural for women but that only certain types of women were encouraged to seek treatment (see Chapters 6 and 7). Young, heterosexual, married, white, affluent women were more likely to be accepted for and able to afford a programme of treatment. Other groups of women who were older, unmarried or lesbian were generally less likely to be offered treatment. This pattern reflects dominant ideas about who should become mothers. NRTs and the new genetics, like other new and emerging health technologies, are deeply embedded within social and cultural processes. While they may have the potential to benefit some women they may also have the potential for harm. The effects of these technologies were seen as complex and sometimes contradictory but never benign.

In the context of new technologies and new knowledge, concepts of health and illness were seen as changing. The development of a genetic approach to health implied a growing emphasis on biological and genetic makeup. At the same time this was seen as having an impact on social relationships and in particular on focusing attention on genetic heritage. Associated with these technologies, distinctions made between social, genetic and legal parents pointed to a rupture in traditional ideas about families and identities. However, we saw how, through legal and policy measures and health care practices, the idea of 'a family' was reasserted alongside individual responsibility. I suggested that increasingly 'mothers' are under pressure to produce healthy babies, while the responsibilities of 'fathers' (including absent ones) continue to be defined primarily in terms of being breadwinners, even though many households depend on mothers working. Values of individualism and an emphasis on the biological (genetic) causes of ill-health characterized contemporary developments in reproductive health.

However, the work of feminist writers, philosophers, artists and photographers was seen as pointing to the ways in which women resist definition and containment. Women's bodies were seen as sites of struggle. The pregnant body was seen as representing a challenge to conventional ideas about individuals as autonomous and separate beings. In pregnancy the boundaries between inside and outside were seen as blurred, with one being attached to another. While the idea of the foetus as a separate subject was criticized in debates around abortion (Petchesky 1987), the emphasis on connection pointed to alternative notions of feminine subjectivity. The 'leakiness' of women's bodies also symbolically undermined traditional ideas of a unitary identity with clearly defined bodily boundaries. Pregnancy, rather than the fulfilment of 'real women', was seen as a paradigmatic case of split subjectivity and fragmentation (see Chapter 8).

In effect such a view of pregnancy and childbirth implies a rethinking of what it means to become a mother. For health care practitioners this means thinking through the view we have of women (and their bodies) seeking maternity care. While in the past the biological and physiological effects of pregnancy and childbirth have been emphasized these discourses have incorporated particular ideas about bodies. The body as machine or as a set of systems with inputs and outputs have been dominant metaphors (Martin 1993). This biomedical model of pregnancy and childbirth has underplayed the social aspects or incorporated these within the model. What I have argued for here is a broader and deeper analysis of the social dimension. Rather than seeing them as separate spheres the biological and the social are deeply intertwined. Bodies are not simply the biological base to social action or acted upon by social processes. Bodies are produced or constituted *by* social processes.

As new types of educational programme for nurses and midwives continue to develop, the expectation is that these practitioners will produce research that informs and improves practice. If this research is to tackle the complex social issues which impact on the lives of women using maternity services and shape their experience of becoming mothers, there is an urgent need to develop a sociological perspective on pregnancy and childbirth. This means engaging with quite complex theoretical debate and developing an understanding of different methodologies (Abbott and Sapsford 1992, 1997). My hope is that this book will, in a small way, contribute to such a project.

Summary

The key themes and ideas running through this book are:

● Pregnancy and childbirth are not simply natural or biological events but are embodied practices that combine both biological and social processes.

● Women's experiences of their bodies, and of pregnancy and childbirth, are socially constructed and culturally mediated.

● The role of health care practitioners such as midwives and nurses may be understood in terms of a particular historical and social context.

- Midwifery knowledge, like other forms of knowledge, is not neutral but is linked to the exercise of power.

- Knowledge and power both regulate and produce bodies and identities.

- Identities are not stable or fixed, but are constantly being negotiated through the discursive ordering of the social world.

- Women are not all the same and the subject 'woman' obscures important differences between women.

- Acknowledging difference means recognizing and responding positively to the different health care needs of women during pregnancy and childbirth.

- Important differences between the 'expert' practitioner and service user also need to be acknowledged and understood if care is to be delivered in equitable ways.

- There are always alternative ways of seeing and doing things and health care practitioners need to be open to these possibilities.

- Being reflexive means recognizing the ways in which health care practitioners' own knowledge and practice is socially and culturally produced.

GLOSSARY

Accounting practices: the ways in which knowledge or discourse is constructed in accounts.

Agency: the ability of individuals to act as agents and reproduce social structures.

Alienation: the separation and distance between a subject and object; a woman and her body treated as an object.

Autonomy: the separation and independence of one individual from others.

Biological determinism: the idea or belief that social phenomena or processes arise directly from biological phenomena or processes.

Biological reductionism: the reduction of all social processes to biological ones.

Bureaucratization: the process of increasing bureaucracy associated with modern societies.

Capitalism: political and economic relationships shaped by the unequal ownership of the means of production (property).

Civilizing process: this describes the historical process of 'civilizing' social behaviour.

Commodification: the process of treating all things as objects which may be bought, sold or exchanged.

Constructionism: the process whereby knowledge is socially constructed.

Corporeal: bodily, physical, material.

Credentialism: the process whereby a professional group seeks to obtain status by the acquisition of formal credentials and qualifications.

Deconstruction: a method of analysing or unpacking how knowledge, discourses or representations are constructed.

Dependency culture: a generally negative view of the need for social support.

Discourses: the linguistic practices and social relationships which construct knowledge.

Division of labour: the dividing of tasks, work and responsibilities between individuals or social groups.

Dual closure: a dual strategy of defending occupational territory or boundaries.

Dual systems approach: an analysis of both patriarchy and capitalism.

Dystopic: the opposite of utopic, a negative and pessimistic view of the future.

Embody (embodiment): to take on a bodily form.

Epistemology: theory of knowledge.

Essentialism: the view that there is a biological basis to sexual and gender identities.

Eugenics: a doctrine about ways of improving the human race through selective breeding.

Experiential knowledge: knowledge based on experience.

Familialism: the ideology of the family, or set of normative values associated with nuclear family life.

Foundationalism: a philosophical view that knowledge is founded, or based on, being – the experiences of being human.

Gender differences: the social divisions between men and women.

Gender relations: relations between men and women.

Hegemonic masculinity: the dominant values, beliefs and ideas of a traditional form of masculinity usually associated with white, middle-class men.

Hegemony: dominant rule or belief.

Heterosexism: discrimination conscious or unconscious, based on the assumption that heterosexuality is 'normal'.

Homogenous: the same or similar.

Homophobia: fear of homosexuality and lesbian sexuality which leads to negative discrimination.

Homophobic: a person who is afraid of, or who discriminates against, homosexuals and/or lesbians.

Horizontal occupational segregation: segregation of jobs which are in a non-hierarchical relationship to each other.

Human capital: the value attributed to knowledge and skills.

Identity politics: a political strategy which rests on the identification of individuals as the same or different from others.

Ideology: a set of beliefs or knowledge used to justify a political position.

Independent variable: an element or phenomenon which is regarded as independent of other factors which may be manipulated to determine its effect upon a 'dependent' variable.

Labour process: the organization of labour, materials and technology.

Marginalization: the effects of discrimination which undervalues individuals or social groups and sees them as peripheral or unimportant.

Masculinist: a culture where masculine values dominate.

Material: the physical or organic.

Material deprivation: poverty, deprivation of material resources.

Materiality: the material or real.

Maternal bonding: the term often used to describe a healthy relationship between a mother and child.

Maternal deprivation: a concept associated with Bowlby's theories of childcare which refers to the negative effects of a child's separation from its mother.

Maternal instinct: the notion that women have a 'natural' motherly instinct (see Biological determinism).

Mechanistic: machine-like.

Medicalization: the use of medical concepts and theories.

Methodological individualism: emphasis on the individual as a unit of analysis.

Modernism: a term to describe the modern era frequently characterized as a period where science, rationality and democracy are key values.

Modernity: the historical development of modern society.

Objectification: treating like an object.

Occupational closure: restricting entry to an occupation.

Occupational segregation: different types of jobs for different types of people, usually refers to segregation of women and men into different types of jobs.

Ontology: branch of metaphysics dealing with the nature of being.

Panopticism: literally means 'seeing everything' but Foucault used the term to describe a type of surveillance classically identified with the structure of a Victorian prison or hospital.

Paradigms: a model of the world, a set of beliefs or theories which shape how the world is viewed.

Patriarchal: see patriarchy.

Patriarchy: a system of oppression and inequality characterized by men having higher social status and power than women.

Phallocentric culture: a culture where the symbol of the phallus is dominant.

Phenomenology: a methodological approach to understanding the social world which focuses on the experiences and understandings of persons.

Polymorphous: of a variety of shapes.

Postmodern: a much contested concept which may be taken to refer to a historical period after modernity but also to the view that social relations are not reducible to fixed subject positions. Rather, subjectivity is seen as discursively produced and constantly being negotiated.

Poststructuralism: the idea that social structures are not fixed. Poststructuralism emphasizes the idea of social relations as dynamic and changing.

Professionalization: the process whereby occupational groups obtain status, the ability to be self-regulating and claim a distinct knowledge base.

Pronatalism: promoting pregnancy and birth for women.

Propositional knowledge: theoretical knowledge based on systematic propositions.

Randomized controlled trials: an experimental research method where subjects are randomly selected and assigned to either an intervention or control group.

Rationalist: rational.

Rationalization: the process of rationalizing, seen as widespread in modern societies.

Reductionism: reducing complex processes to single or simple units of analysis.

Representations: the symbols or images used to stand for something else.

Scientific paradigm: the scientific model characterized by an emphasis on observable, measureable phenomena.

Scientization: the growth and extension of scientific forms of reasoning and knowledge.

Secularization: the decline of religion and religious beliefs in the modern world and the tendency to become a secular society.

Sex differences: biological differences between male and female.

Sexology: the scientific study of sex.

Sexual division of labour: a separation of tasks defined as either women's work or men's work.

Sexual identity: the social construction of an identity related to sexual practice.

Sexual politics: the ways in which power shapes sexual relations.

Social constructionism: the ways in which social processes shape or influence ideas, knowledge and beliefs.

Social exclusion: marginalization from mainstream social life, lacking in power and status.

Social integration: part of a social collectivity. Systems and institutional structures develop to create relative harmony between different social groups.

Social norms: socially accepted ways of behaving.

Socialization: the process of becoming socialized, through learnt behaviour and attitudes.

Stigmatization: a negative labelling of an individual or social group.

Stereotype: the attribution of negative characteristics to a specific individual based on their membership of a group.

Stratification theory: theory which explains social divisions and inequalities in society in terms of a tiered and hierarchical organization.

Surveillance: the regulation, discipline and control of bodies or populations by observational methods.

Symbolism: the construction of meaning using symbols and signs, for example language.

Technical rationality: a type of reasoning and knowledge which is orientated towards technological definitions and solutions of problems.

Technologically determinist: social relationships seen as arising directly from specific technologies.

Universalism: the principle that theories or results may be applied across populations and cultures – that is, universally.

Vertical occupational segregation: segregation of jobs in an hierarchical order.

REFERENCES

Abbott, P. and Sapsford, R. (1992) *Research Methods for Nurses and the Caring Professions*. Buckingham: Open University Press.

Abbott, P. and Sapsford, R. (eds) (1997) *Research into Practice: A Reader for Nurses and the Caring Professions*. Buckingham: Open University Press.

Abbott, P. and Wallace, C. (eds) (1990) *The Sociology of the Caring Professions*. Basingstoke: Falmer Press.

Abramsky, L. (1994) Counselling prior to prenatal testing, in L. Abramsky and J. Chapple (eds) *Prenatal Diagnosis: The Human Side*. London: Chapman & Hall.

Ackerman, B. and Winkler, L. (1979) Briggs, the Bill and the new clause, *ARM Newsletter*, February: 5–7.

Ackers, L. and Abbott, P. (1996) *Social Policy for Nurses and the Caring Professions*. Buckingham: Open University Press.

Adams, A. (1994) *Reproducing the Womb: Images of Childbirth in Science, Feminist Theory and Literature*. London: Cornell University Press.

Adkins, L. (1995) *Gendered Work: Sexuality, Family and the Labour Market*. Buckingham: Open University Press.

Alcoff, L. and Potter, E. (eds) (1993) *Feminist Epistemologies*. London: Routledge.

Annandale, E. (1988) How midwives accomplish natural birth: managing risk and balancing expectations, *Social Problems*, 35(2): 95–110.

Annandale, E. (1998) *The Sociology of Health & Medicine: A Critical Introduction*. Oxford: Polity Press.

Annandale, E. and Clark, J. (1996) What is gender? Feminist theory and the sociology of human reproduction, *Sociology of Health & Illness*, 18(1): 17–44.

Arditti, R., Klein, R. and Minden, S. (1984) *Test-tube Women: What Future for Motherhood?* London: Pandora.

Asch, A. and Fine, M. (1997) Nurturance, sexuality and women with disabilities, in L. Davis (ed.) *The Disability Studies Reader*. London: Routledge.

Assister, A. (1996) *Enlightened Women: Modernist Feminism in a Post-Modern Age*. London: Routlege.

Association of Radical Midwives (1980) Direct entry: three experiences, *Association of Radical Midwives Newsletter*, 8(October): 6–7.

Association Radical Midwives (1981) Direct entry training, *Association of Radical Midwives Newsletter*, 9(February): 17.

Association Radical Midwives (1986) Direct entry training, *Association of Radical Midwives Newsletter*, 28.

Bahvnami, K. (1997) Women's studies and its interconnection with 'race', ethnicity and sexuality, in V. Robinson and D. Richardson (eds) *Introducing Women's Studies*, 2nd edn. London: Macmillan.

Ball, H. (1982) Direct entrant midwives: a special class, *Midwives Chronicle and Nursing Notes*, January.

Barron, R. and Norris, G. (1976) Sexual divisions and the dual labour market, in L. Barker and S. Allen (eds) *Dependence and Exploitation in Work and Marriage*. London: Longman.

BBC (1997) *Timewatch: Birth Story, Fifty Years of Childbirth*, 25 March.

Beck, U. (1992) *Risk Society Towards a New Modernity*. London: Sage.

Becker, H., Geer, B., Hughs, E. and Strauss, L. (1961) *Boys in White*. Chicago: University of Chicago Press.

Benn, M. (1998) *Madonna and Child: Towards a New Politics of Motherhood*. London: Jonathan Cape.

Benoit, C. (1989) The professional socialisation of midwives: balancing art and science, *Sociology of Health and Illness*, 11(2): 160–80.

Bephage, G. (1997) *Social Science and Healthcare: Nursing Applications in Clinical Practice*. London: Mosby.

Berryman, J. (1991) Perspectives on later motherhood, in A. Phoenix, A. Woollett and E. Lloyd (eds) *Motherhood: Meanings, Practices and Ideologies*. London: Sage.

Berryman, J. and Windridge, K. (1995) *Motherhood After 35: A Report on the Leicester Motherhood Project*. Leicester: University of Leicester.

Berryman, J., Thorpe, K. and Windridge, K. (1995) *Older Mothers: Conception, Pregnancy and Birth After 35*. London: Pandora, HarperCollins.

Betterton, R. (1996) *An Intimate Distance: Women, Artists and the Body*. London: Routledge.

Bonner, F., Goodman, L., Allen, R., Janes, L. and King, C. (eds) (1992) *Imagining Women: Cultural Representations and Gender*. Cambridge: Polity Press.

Bordo, S. (1995) *Unbearable Weight, Feminism: Western Culture and the Body*. Berkeley, CA: University of California Press.

Bortolaia Silva, E. (ed.) (1996) *Good Enough Mothering? Feminist Perspectives on Lone Motherhood*. London: Routledge.

Borzello, F. (1998) *Seeing Ourselves: Women's Self-Portraits*. London: Thames & Hudson.

Bowlby, R. (1993) *Shopping With Freud*. London: Routledge.

Bradley, H. (1989) *Men's Work: Women's Work*. Cambridge: Polity Press.

Brannen, J. and Moss, P. (1988) *New Mothers at Work: Employment and Childcare*. London: Unwin Hyman.

Brannen, J. and Moss, P. (1990) *Managing Mothers: Employment and Childcare*. London: Unwin Hyman.

Brien, J. and Fairbairn, I. (1996) *Pregnancy and Abortion Counselling*. London: Routledge.

Brogan, M. (1997) Healthcare for lesbians: attitudes and experiences, *Nursing Standard*, 11(45): 39–42.

Bruegel, I. (1979) Women as a reserve army of labour: a note on recent British experience, *Feminist Review*, 3: 12–23.

Bryar, R. (1995) *Theory for Midwifery Practice*. London: Macmillan.

Bryson, A., Ford, R. and White, M. (1997) *Making Work Pay: Lone Mothers, Employment and Well-being*. York: Joseph Rowntree Foundation.

Burdet, C. (1996) Cell-by date for embryos, *Bath Chronicle*, 25 July: 27.

Burgess, A. and Ruxton, S. (1996) *Men and Their Children: Proposals for Public Policy*. London: Institute for Public Policy Research.

Busfield, J. (1996) *Men, Women and Madness: Understanding Gender and Mental Disorder*. London: Macmillan.

Buswell, C. (1992) Training girls to be low-paid women, in C. Glendinning and J. Millar (eds) *Women and Poverty in Britain in the 1990s*. Hemel Hempstead: Harvester Wheatsheaf.

Butler, J. (1990) *Gender Trouble: Feminism and the Subversion of Identity*. London: Routlege.

Butler, J. (1993) *Bodies That Matter: On the Discursive Limits of Sex*. London: Routledge.

Buurman, G. (1997) Erotic bodies: images of the disabled, in K. Davis (ed.) *Embodied Practices*. London: Sage.

Callahan, J. (ed.) (1995) *Reproduction, Ethics and the Law: Feminist Perspectives*. Bloomington, IN: Indiana University Press.

Campbell, R. and Mcfarlane, A. (1990) Recent debate on the place of birth, in J. Garcia, R. Fitzpatrick and M. Richards (eds) *The Politics of Maternity Care: Services for Childbearing Women in Twentieth-Century Britain.* Oxford: Oxford University Press.

Campbell, R. and Macfarlane, A. (1994) *Where to be Born? The Debate and the Evidence,* 2nd edn. Oxford: National Perinatal Epidemiology Unit.

Campbell, R. and Porter, S. (1997) Feminist theory and the sociology of childbirth: a response to Ellen Annandale and Judith Clark, *Sociology of Health & Illness,* 19(3): 348–58.

Cardale, P. (1990) Breaking away, *Nursing Times,* 86(28): 68–9.

Chadwick, R. (1990) The perfect baby, in R. Chadwick (ed.) *Ethics, Reproduction and Genetic Control.* London: Routledge.

Chandler, J. (1991) *Women Without Husbands: An Exploration of the Margins of Marriage.* London: Macmillan.

Chapman, C. (1992) *Theory of Nursing: Practical Application.* London: Harper & Row.

Chodorow, N. (1978) *The Reproduction of Mothering: Psychoanalysis and the Sociology of Gender.* Berkeley, CA: University of California Press.

Clarke, A. (1991) Is non-directive genetic counselling possible? *Lancet,* 338: 998–1000.

Clarke, A. (ed.) (1994) *Genetic Counselling Practice and Principles.* London: Routledge.

Cockburn, C. (1983) *Brothers: Male Dominance and Technological Change.* London: Pluto Press.

Cockburn, C. (1985) *Machinery of Dominance: Women, Men and Technical Knowhow.* London: Pluto Press.

Collins, H. (1985) *Changing Order: Replication and Induction in Scientific Practice.* London: Sage.

Collins, P. (1993) Black feminist thought, in S. Jackson, K. Atkinson, D. Beddoe *et al.* (eds) *Women's Studies: A Reader.* Hemel Hempstead: Harvester Wheatsheaf.

Connell, R. (1987) *Gender and Power: Society, the Person and Sexual Politics.* Cambridge: Polity Press.

Connell, R. (1995) *Masculinities.* Cambridge: Polity Press.

Cook, J. and Watt, S. (1992) Racism, women and poverty, in C. Glendinning and J. Millar (eds) *Women and Poverty in Britain in the 1990s.* Hemel Hempstead: Harvester Wheatsheaf.

Corea, G. (1985) *Man-made Women.* London: Hutchinson.

Coufopoulos, A. and Stitt, S. (1994) 'Teenage mums, the "underclass" and sex education', unpublished paper presented at British Sociological Association Annual Conference, University of Central Lancashire.

Cox, D. (1991) Health service management – a sociological view: Griffiths and the non-negotiated order of the hospital, in J. Gabe, M. Calnan and M. Bury (eds) *The Sociology of the Health Service.* London: Routledge.

Crompton, R. (1990) Class theory and gender, *The British Journal of Sociology,* 40(4): 565–86.

Crompton, R. and Mann, M. (eds) (1986) *Gender and Stratification.* Cambridge: Polity Press.

Crompton, R. and Sanderson, K. (1990) *Gendered Jobs and Social Change.* London: Unwin Hyman.

Cronk, M. (1990) Midwifery: a practitioner's view from within the National Health Service, *Midwife, Health Visitor and Community Nurse,* 26(3): 58, 61, 63.

Curtis, P. (1986) 'Direct entry into midwifery: some implications for independent practitioner status', unpublished dissertation. University of Leeds.

Dalley, G. (1988) *Ideologies of Caring.* London: Macmillan.

Dallos, R. and Sapsford, R. (1995) Patterns of diversity and lived realities, in J. Muncie, M. Wetherell, R. Dallos and A. Cochrane (eds) *Understanding the Family.* London: Sage.

Dally, A. (1982) *Inventing Motherhood: The Consequences of an Ideal.* London: Hutchinson.

Dalmiya, V. and Alcoff, L. (1993) Are 'old wives' tales' justified?, in L. Alcoff and E. Potter (eds) *Feminist Epistemologies*. London: Routledge.

Darke, G. (1996) Discourses on the menopause and female sexuality, in J. Holland and L. Adkins (eds) *Sex, Sensibility and the Gendered Body*. London: Macmillan.

Darke, G. and Kent, J. (forthcoming) Changing fortune: the corporeal limits to reflexivity, unpublished paper.

Davies, C. (1995) *Gender and the Professional Predicament in Nursing*. Buckingham: Open University Press.

Davies, R. and Atkinson, P. (1991) Students of midwifery: doing the obs and other coping strategies, *Midwifery*, 7: 113–21.

Davis, K. (ed.) (1997) *Embodied Practices: Feminist Perspectives on the Body*. London: Sage.

Davison, C., Macintyre, S. and Davey Smith, G. (1994) The potential impact of predictive genetic testing for susceptibility to common chronic diseases: a review and proposed research agenda, *Sociology of Health & Illness*, 16(3): 340–71.

Department of Health (1979) *Nurses, Midwives and Health Visitors Act*. London: HMSO.

Department of Health (1989a) *Review of the Guidance on the Research Use of Fetuses and Fetal Material*. London: HMSO.

Department of Health (1989b) *Working for Patients: Education and Training Working Paper 10*. London: HMSO.

Department of Health (1990) *Human Fertilisation and Embryology Act*. London: HMSO.

Department of Health (1992) *NHS Workforce in England, 1982–1992*. London: HMSO.

Department of Health (1993) *Changing Childbirth, Part 1: Report of the Expert Maternity Group*. London: HMSO.

Department of Health (1995) *Improving the Health of the Mothers and Children: NHS Priorities for Research and Development*. Leeds: Department of Health.

Department of Trade & Industry (DTI) (1997) *Human Genetics Advisory Commission*. London: DTI.

DeVault, M. (1991) *Feeding the Family: The Social Organisation of Caring as Gendered Work*. London: University of Chicago Press.

Devries, R. (1982) Midwifery and the problem of licensure in research, *The Sociology of Health Care*, 2: 77–129.

Dex, S. (1988) *Women's Attitudes Towards Work*. Basingstoke: Macmillan.

Dickson, N. (1986) Begging to differ, *Nursing Times*, 82(28): 67–70.

Dillner, L. (1996a) Ethics at issue, *Guardian*, 27 August.

Dillner, L. (1996b) Woman could die bearing octuplets, *Guardian*, 12 August.

Dingwall, R. (1977) *The Social Organization of Health Visiting*. London: Croom Helm.

Dingwall, R. and Lewis, P. (eds) (1983) *The Sociology of Professions*. London: Macmillan.

Donnison, J. (1977) *Midwives and Medical Men: A History of Interprofessional Rivalries*. London: Schocken Books.

Douglas, J. (1998) Meeting the health needs of women from black and minority ethnic communities, in L. Doyal (ed.) *Women and Health Services*. Buckingham: Open University Press.

Downe, S. (1986a) Direct entry working party, *ARM Newsletter*, 29: 49–50.

Downe, S. (1986b) Dispelling the myths on direct entry training, *Nursing Times*, 82(37): 63–4.

Downe, S. (1987) Direct entry midwifery training: the future for English midwifery? in *MIDIRS Information Pack*. Bristol: MIDIRS.

Downe, S. (1990) Midwives stand alone, *Nursing Times*, 86(24): 22.

Downe, S. (1991) Who defines abnormality? *Nursing Times*, 87(18): 22.

Doyal, L. (1987) Infertility, a life sentence? Women and the National Health Service, in M. Stanworth (ed.) *Reproductive Technologies: Gender, Motherhood and Medicine*. Oxford: Basil Blackwell.

Doyal, L. (1994) Changing medicine? Gender and the politics of health care, in M. Gabe, D. Kelleher and G. Williams (eds) *Challenging Medicine*, 2nd edn. London: Routledge.

Doyal, L. (1995) *What Makes Women Sick? Gender and the Political Economy of Health*. London: Macmillan.

Doyal, L. (ed.) (1998) *Women and Health Services*. Buckingham: Open University Press.

Dreyfus, H. and Rabinow, P. (1982) *Michel Foucault: Beyond Structuralism and Hermeneutics*. Brighton: Harvester.

Dunkerley, D. and Glasner, P. (1998) Empowering the public? Citizens' juries and the new genetic technologies, *Critical Public Health*, 8(3): 181–92.

Durward, L. and Evans, R. (1990) Pressure groups and maternity care, in J. Garcia, R. Fitzpatrick and M. Richards (eds) *The Politics of Maternity Care: Services for Childbearing Women in Twentieth-Century Britain*. Oxford: Oxford University Press.

Dyer, C., Bosely, S. and Radford, T. (1996) How ethics and the law joined a fight for new life after death, *Guardian*, 23 November: 3.

Edley, N. and Wetherell, M. (1995) *Men in Perspective, Practice: Power and Identity*. London: Prentice Hall.

EEC (European Economic Community) (1980) *Midwives Directives 80/154/EEC and 80/155/EEC*. Brussels: EEC.

Elston, M. (1991) The politics of professional power: medicine in a changing health service, in J. Gabe, M. Calnan and M. Bury (eds) *The Sociology of the Health Service*. London: Routledge.

ENB (English National Board for Nursing, Midwifery and Health Visiting) (1985) *Proposals for Change*. London: ENB.

ENB (English National Board for Nursing, Midwifery and Health Visiting) (1990) *Regulations and Guidelines for Approval of Institutions and Courses 1990*. London: ENB.

ENB (English National Board for Nursing, Midwifery and Health Visiting) (1992) *Approved Midwife Teacher, ENB Circular 1992/04/PAA*. London: ENB.

ENB (English National Board for Nursing, Midwifery and Health Visiting) (1993a) *Regulations and Guidelines for the Approval of Institutions and Courses 1993*. London: ENB.

ENB (English National Board for Nursing, Midwifery and Health Visiting) (1993b) *Integrating Nursing and Midwifery Education into Higher Education: A Good Practice Guide*. London: ENB.

ENB (English National Board for Nursing, Midwifery and Health Visiting) (1997) Research highlights at http://www.enb.org.uk

ENB (English National Board for Nursing, Midwifery and Health Visiting) (1998a) *The Regulation of Nurses, Midwives and Health Visitors: Response of the English National Board*. London: ENB.

ENB (English National Board for Nursing, Midwifery and Health Visiting) (1998b) Developments in the use of an evidence and/or enquiry based approach in nursing, midwifery and health visiting programmes of educationat at http://www.enb.org.uk

Eraut, M., Alderton, J., Boylan, A. and Wraight, A. (1995) *Learning to Use Scientific Knowledge in Education and Practice Settings: An Evaluation of the Contribution of the Biological Behavioural and Social Sciences to Pre-registration Nursing and Midwifery Programmes*. London: ENB.

Everingham, C. (1994) *Motherhood and Modernity*. Buckingham: Open University Press.

Farquhar, D. (1996) *The Other Machine: Discourse and Reproductive Technologies*. London: Routledge.

Faugier, J. (1994) Bad women and good customers: scapegoating female prostitution and HIV, in C. Webb (ed.) *Living Sexuality: Issues for Nursing and Health.* Harrow: Scutari.

Ferguson, K. (1993) *The Man Question: Visions of Subjectivity in Feminist Theory.* Berkeley, CA: University of California Press.

Ferguson, K. (1994) Mental health and sexuality, in C. Webb (ed.) *Living Sexuality: Issues for Nursing and Health.* Harrow: Scutari.

Finch, J. and Groves, D. (eds) (1983) *A Labour of Love: Women, Work and Caring.* London: Routledge and Kegan Paul.

Flint, C. (1986) Should midwives train as florists?, *Nursing Times*, 82(7): 21.

Flint, C. (1997) Midwives will carry the can, *Midwives Journal*, 110(1311): 96.

Flint, C. and Poulengerie, P. (1991) *The Know Your Midwife Report.* Bristol: MIDIRS.

Foucault, M. (1973) *The Birth of the Clinic: An Archaeology of Medical Perception.* London: Tavistock.

Foucault, M. (1979) *The History of Sexuality, Vol. 1: An Introduction.* Harmondsworth: Penguin.

Foucault, M. (1985) *The History of Sexuality, Vol. 2: The Use of Pleasure.* Harmondsworth: Penguin.

Foucault, M. (1990) *The History of Sexuality, Vol. 3: The Care of the Self.* Harmondsworth: Penguin.

Frame, S. and North, J. (1990) 'Will History Repeat itself?' *ARM Midwifery Matters*, 44: 6–7.

Frank, A. (1991a) For a sociology of the body, in M. Featherstone, M. Hepworth, and M. Turner (eds) *The Body: Social Process and Cultural Theory.* London: Sage.

Frank, A. (1991b) *At the Will of the Body: Reflections on Illness.* Boston, MA: Houghton Mifflin.

Frank, A. (1996) Reconciliatory alchemy: bodies, narratives and power, *Body & Society*, 2(3): 53–71.

Franklin, S. (1997) *Embodied Progress: A Cultural Account of Assisted Conception.* London: Routledge.

Fraser, D., Murphy, R. and Worth-Butler, M. (1997) *An Outcome Evaluation of the Effectiveness of Pre-registration Midwifery Programmes of Education.* London: ENB.

Freud, S. (1961) *The Standard Edition of the Complete Psychological Works of Sigmund Freud, vol. 11 (1927–1931)* (trans. J. Strachey). London: Hogarth Press.

Freud, S. (1986) *On Sexuality: Three Essays on the Theory of Sexuality and Other Works.* Harmondsworth: Penguin.

Fuss, D. (1989) *Essentially Speaking: Feminism, Nature and Difference.* London: Routledge.

Gabe, J., Kelleher, D. and Williams, G. (eds) (1994) *Challenging Medicine.* London: Routledge.

Gallop, J. (1988) *Thinking Through the Body.* Oxford: Columbia University Press.

Garcia, J., Kilpatrick, R. and Richards, M. (eds) (1990) *The Politics of Maternity Care Services for Childbearing Women in the Twentieth Century.* Oxford: Clarendon Press.

Gardiner, J. (1997) *Gender Care and Economics.* London: Macmillan.

Gatens, M. (1996) *Imaginary Bodies: Ethics, Power and Corporeality.* London: Routledge.

Gaze, H. (1987) Men in Nursing, *Nursing Times*, 83(20): 25–7.

Genetic Interest Group (1998) *Annual Report 1997/98.* London: GIG.

Gerrish, K., Husband, C. and Mackenzie, J. (1996a) *An Examination of the Extent to which Pre-registration Programmes of Nursing and Midwifery Prepare Practitioners to Meet the Health Needs of Minority Ethnic Communities.* London: ENB.

Gerrish, K., Husband, C. and Mackenzie, J. (1996b) *Nursing for a Multi-Ethnic Society.* Buckingham: Open University Press.

Giddens, A. (1991) *Modernity and Self Identity.* Cambridge: Polity Press.

Gilligan, C. (1982) *In a Different Voice: Psychological Theory and Women's Development.* London: Harvard University Press.

Gilman, S. (1985) Black bodies, white bodies: towards an iconography of female sexuality in the late nineteenth century, *Critical Inquiry* 12(1): 205–43.

Gittins, D. (1985) *The Family Question: Changing Households and Familiar Ideologies*. London: Macmillan.

Glendinning, C. and Millar, J. (eds) (1992) *Women and Poverty in Britain in the 1990s*. Hemel Hempstead: Harvester Wheatsheaf.

Gordon, S. (1991) *The History and Philosophy of Social Science*. London: Routledge.

Gordon, T. (1990) *Feminist Mothers*. London: Macmillan.

Gordon, T. (1994) *Single Women*. London: Macmillan.

Graham, H. (1983) Caring: a labour of love, in J. Finch and D. Groves (eds) *A Labour of Love: Women, Work and Caring*. London: Routledge and Kegan Paul.

Graham, H. (1991) The concept of caring in feminist research: the case of domestic service, *Sociology*, 25(1): 61–78.

Graham, H. (1992) Budgeting for health: mothers in low income households, in C. Glendinning and J. Millar (eds) *Women and Poverty in Britain in the 1990s*. Hemel Hempstead: Harvester Wheatsheaf.

Gready, M. *et al*. (1995) *Birth Choices: Women's Expectations and Experiences of a Research Project: Childbirth Options Information and Care in Essex*. London: National Childbirth Trust.

Green, J. (1990) Calming or harming: a critical review of psychological effects of fetal diagnosis on pregnant women, *Galton Institute Occasional Papers, second series, no. 2*.

Green, J. (1994) Women's experiences of screening and diagnosis, in L. Abramsky and J. Chapple (eds) *Prenatal Diagnosis: The Human Side*. London: Chapman & Hall.

Grosz, E. (1995) *Space, Time and Perversion: Essays on the Politics of Bodies*. London: Routledge.

Groves, D. (1992) Occupational pension provision and women's poverty in old age, in C. Glendinning and J. Millar (eds) *Women and Poverty in Britain in the 1990s*. Hemel Hempstead: Harvester Wheatsheaf.

Guardian (1996) Can a widow be a mother? 1 October.

Hahn, H. (1983) Paternalism and public policy, *Society*, March–April: 36–44.

Hall, S. (1992) The question of cultural identity, in S. Hall, D. Held and T. McGrew (eds) *Modernity and Its Futures*. Cambridge: Polity Press.

Hall, S. (1997a) *Representation: Cultural Representations and Signifying Practices*. London: Sage.

Hall, S. (1997b) The spectacle of the 'Other', in S. Hall (ed.) *Representation: Cultural Representations and Signifying Practices*. London: Sage.

Hansard (1996) House of Commons science policy and human genetics debate, 19 July, pp. 1409–82.

Hansch, A. (1997) The body of the woman artist, *The European Journal of Women's Studies*, 4(4): 435–49.

Haraway, D. (1991) *Simians, Cyborgs and Women: The Reinvention of Nature*. London: Free Association Books.

Harding, S. (1986) *The Science Question in Feminism*. Milton Keynes: Open University Press.

Harding, S. (1991) *Whose Science? Whose Knowledge? Thinking from Women's Lives*. Buckingham: Open University Press.

Harding, S. (1993) Rethinking standpoint theory: what is strong objectivity? in L. Alcoff and E. Potter (eds) *Feminist Epistemologies*. London: Routledge.

Harrison, B. (1995) Every picture tells a story: uses of the visual in sociological research. Paper presented at British Sociological Association Annual Conference 'Research Imaginations', University of Essex.

Harrison, B. and Aranda, K. (1997) Power, photography and medicine, in E. Stina Lyon and J. Busfield (eds) *Methodological Imaginations*. Basingstoke: Macmillan.

Hartmann, H. (1979) Capitalism, patriarchy and job segregation by sex, in Z. Eisenstein (ed.) *Capitalist Patriarchy and the Case for Socialist Feminism*. New York: Monthly Review Press.

Hartmann, H. (1981) The unhappy marriage of Marxism and feminism: towards a more progressive union, in A. Sassoon (ed.) *Women and Revolution*. New York: Monthly Review Press.

Hatt, S. (1997) *Gender Work and Labour Markets*. London: Macmillan.

Hawkes, G. (1996) *A Sociology of Sex and Sexuality*. Buckingham: Open University Press.

Health Education Authority (1994) *Sexual Health*. London: Health Education Authority.

Health Technology Assessment (1995) at http://www.hta.nhsweb.nhs.uk

Hearn, J. (1987) *The Gender of Oppression*. Brighton: Harvester Wheatsheaf.

Hekman, S. (1990) *Gender and Knowledge: Elements of a Postmodern Feminism*. Cambridge: Polity Press.

Henderson, C. (1990) Models and midwifery, in J. Salvage and B. Kershaw (eds) *Models for Nursing 2*. Harrow: Scutari.

Henderson, C. (1994) The education and training of midwives, in G. Chamberlain and N. Patel (eds) *The Future of Maternity Services*. London: Royal College of Obstetricians and Gynaecologists.

Hewison, J. and Dowswell, T. (1994) *Child Health Care and the Working Mother: 'The Juggling Act'*. London: Chapman & Hall.

HFEA (Human Fertilisation and Embryology Authority) (1995) *Sperm and Egg Donors and the Law*. London: HFEA.

HFEA (Human Fertilisation and Embryology Authority) (1997) *The Patients' Guide to DI and IVF Clinics*, 3rd edn. London: HFEA.

Ho, E. (1991) Changes in midwifery education, for better or for worse, *Midwifery Matters*, 49: 4.

Hollway, W. and Featherstone, B. (eds) (1997) *Mothering and Ambivalence*. London: Routledge.

Hooper, C. (1997) 'Manly states: masculinities, international relations and gender politics', unpublished PhD thesis. University of Bristol.

House of Commons Select Committee (1992) *Second Report: Maternity Services*. London: HMSO.

Hubbard, R. (1997) Abortion and disability, in L. Davis (ed.) *The Disability Studies Reader*. London: Routledge.

Hughes, D. and Parker, O. (1986) Training for the future, *Nursing Times*, 82(37): 51–62.

Hugman, P. (1991) *Power in the Caring Professions*. London: Macmillan.

Hunt, S. and Symonds, A. (1995) *The Social Meaning of Midwifery*. London: Macmillan.

Irigaray, L. (1985a) *Speculum of the Other Woman*. Ithaca, NY: Cornell University Press.

Irigaray, L. (1985b) *This Sex Which is not One*. Ithaca, NY: Cornell University Press.

Irwin, R. (1997) Sexual health promotion and nursing, *Journal of Advanced Nursing*, 25(1): 170–7.

Jackson, K. (1993) Midwifery degree programmes: who benefits? *British Journal of Midwifery* 1(6): 274–5.

Jackson, K. (1995) Changing childbirth: the work of the implementation team, in *Changing Childbirth Educational Resource Pack for Midwives, no. 4, Control in Practice*. London: ENB.

Jackson, S. and Scott, S. (eds) (1996) *Feminism and Sexuality: A Reader*. Edinburgh: Edinburgh University Press.

Jackson, S., Atkinson, K., Beddoe, D. *et al.* (eds) (1993) *Women's Studies: A Reader*. Hemel Hempstead: Harvester Wheatsheaf.

Jacobus, M., Keller, E. and Shuttleworth, S. (eds) (1990) *Body Politics: Women, Literature and the Discourse of Science*. London: Routledge.

Jannke, S. (1996) Teen pregnancy: the roots of the problem (part one), *Childbirth Instructor Magazine* 6(2): 14–16, 37.

Jenkins, R. (1993) The professional midwife. Unpublished paper presented at the Royal College of Midwives Education Conference 'From Utopia to Reality', London.

JM Consulting Ltd (1998) *The Regulation of Nurses, Midwives and Health Visitors: Invitation to Comment on Issues Raised by a Review of the Nurses, Midwives and Health Visitors Act 1997*. Bristol: JM Consulting Ltd.

Jones, L. and Webb, C. (1994) Young men's experiences of testicular cancer, in C. Webb (ed.) *Living Sexuality: Issues for Nursing and Health*. Harrow: Scutari.

Jordan, B. (1983) *Birth in Four Cultures: A Cross-cultural Investigation of Childbirth in Yucata, Holland, Sweden and the United States*, 3rd edn. Montreal: Eden Press.

Joshi, H. (1992) The cost of caring, in C. Glendinning and J. Millar (eds) *Women and Poverty in Britain in the 1990s*. London: Macmillan.

Joshi, H. and Newell, M. (1987) Job downgrading after childbearing, in M. Uncles (ed.) *Longitudinal Data Analysis: Methods & Applications*. London: Pion.

Katz Rothman, B. (1982) *In Labour: Women and Power in the Birth-Place*. London: Junction Books.

Katz Rothman, B. (1994) *The Tentative Pregnancy: Amniocentesis and the Sexual Politics of Motherhood*. London: Pandora.

Kelly, M. (1997) Exploring midwifery knowledge, *British Journal of Midwifery*, 5(4): 195–8.

Kenny, C. (1996) Against her judgement, *Nursing Times*, 92(41): 16–17.

Kent, J. (1995) 'With women, a reflexive project: knowledge and power in midwifery education', unpublished PhD thesis. University of Bristol.

Kent, J. (1999) Constructing accounts of becoming a midwife: a politics of identity, *Self, Agency and Society: A Journal of Applied Sociology*, 2(1): 23–52.

Kent, J., Barnett, B., Koster, A. *et al.* (1992) Research with, not on . . . challenging the scientific model. Paper presented at RCN Annual Conference on Nursing Research 'The Science of Nursing', Swansea University.

Kent, J., MacKeith, N. and Maggs, C. (1994) *Direct But Different: An Evaluation of the Implementation of Pre-Registration Midwifery Education in England*, vols 1 & 2. Bath: Maggs Research Associates.

Kerr, A., Cunningham-Burley, S. and Amos, A. (1997) The new genetics: professionals; discursive boundaries, in *Sociological Review*, 45: 279–303.

Kerr, A., Cunningham-Burley, S. and Amos, A. (1998) The new genetics and health: mobilising lay expertise, *Public Understanding of Science*, 7(1): 41–60.

King, C. (1992) The politics of representation: a democracy of the gaze, in F. Bonner, L. Goodman, R. Allen, L. Janes and C. King (eds) *Imagining Women: Cultural Representations and Gender*. Cambridge: Polity Press.

Kirkham, M. (1983) Labouring in the dark: limitations on giving of information to enable patients to orientate themselves to the likely events and timescale of labour, in J. Wilson-Barnet (ed.) *Nursing Research: Ten Studies in Patient Care*. Chichester: Wiley.

Kirkham, M. (1989) Midwives and information giving during labour, in S. Robinson and A. Thomson (eds) *Midwives, Research and Childbirth*, vol. 1. London: Chapman & Hall.

Kirkham, M. (1996) Professionalization past and present: with women or with the powers that be? in D. Kroll (ed.) *Midwifery Care for the Future: Meeting the Challenge*. London: Bailliere Tindall.

Kitson, A. (1997) Lessons from the 1996 research assessment exercise, *Nurse Researcher*, 4(3): 81–93.

Kitzinger, J. (1990) Strategies of the early childbirth movement: a case-study of the National Childbirth Trust, in J. Garcia, R. Fitzpatrick and M. Richards (eds) *The Politics of Maternity Care: Services for Childbearing Women in Twentieth-Century Britain*. Oxford: Oxford University Press.

Kitzinger, J., Green, J. and Coupland, V. (1990) Labour relations: midwives and doctors on the labour ward, in J. Garcia, R. Fitzpatrick and M. Richards (eds) *The Politics of Maternity Care: Services for Childbearing Women in Twentieth-Century Britain*. Oxford: Oxford University Press.

Kitzinger, S. (ed.) (1988) *The Midwife Challenge*. London: Pandora.

Kitzinger, S. (1989) Childbirth and Society, in I. Chalmers, M. Enkin and M. Keirse (eds) *Effective Care in Pregnancy and Childbirth*, vol. 1. Oxford: Chalmer Press.

Kitzinger, S. (1992) *Ourselves as Mothers*. London: Doubleday.

Klein, R. (1983) *The Politics of the NHS*. London: Longman.

Klein, R. (ed.) (1989) *Infertility: Women Speak Out About Their Experiences of Reproductive Medicine*. London: Pandora.

Koehn, D. (1994) *The Ground of Professional Ethics*. London: Routledge.

Kristeva, J. (1982) *Powers of Horror: An Essay on Abjection* (trans. L. Raudiez). New York: Columbia University Press.

Krum, S. (1998) When 4 into 55 won't go, *Guardian*, 25 August: 4–5.

Kuhn, T. (1970) *The Structure of Scientific Revolutions*. Chicago: University of Chicago Press.

Leap, N. and Hunter, B. (1993) *The Midwife's Tale: An Oral History from Handywoman to Professional Midwife*. London: Scarlet Press.

Leder, D. (1995) *Qualified Nurses, Midwives and Health Visitors: A Survey Carried out by Social Division of Office of Population, Census & Surveys*. London: HMSO.

Lee-Treweek, G. (1997) Women, resistance and care: an ethnographic study of nursing auxillary work, *Work Employment and Society*, 11(1): 47–63.

Lees, S. (1993) *Sugar and Spice: Sexuality and Adolescent Girls*. Harmondsworth: Penguin.

Levitt, M. (1998) *Evaluation of a Public Education Facility*. Preston: University of Central Lancashire.

Lewis, C. (1987) *Becoming a Father*. Milton Keynes: Open University Press.

Lewis, C. and O'Brien, M. (1987) *Reassessing Fatherhood: New Observations on Father and the Modern Family*. London: Sage

Lewis, J. (1980) *The Politics of Motherhood*. London: Croom Helm.

Lewis, J. (1990) Mothers and maternity policies in the twentieth century, in J. Garcia, R. Fitzpatrick and M. Richards (eds) *The Politics of Maternity Care: Services for Childbearing Women in Twentieth-Century Britain*. Oxford: Oxford University Press.

Lewis, J. (1992) Gender and the development of welfare regimes, *Journal of European Social Policy*, 2(3): 159–73.

Lewis, J. and Meredith, B. (1988) *Daughters who Care: Daughters Caring for Mothers at Home*. London: Routledge.

Lewis, P. (1991) Men in midwifery: their experiences as students and as practitioners, in S. Robinson and A. Thomson (eds) *Midwives, Research & Careers*. London: Croom Helm.

Lewis, R. (1997) Insurance for independent midwives, that ongoing saga, in Association Radical Midwives, *Midwifery Matters*, Spring, 72: 6–7.

Littlewood, R. (1991) Gender, role and sickness: the ritual psychopathologies of the nurse, in P. Holden and J. Littlewood (eds) *Anthropology and Nursing*. London: Routledge.

Lonsdale, S. (1990) *Women and Disability: The Experience of Physical Disability Among Women*. London: Macmillan.

Lupton, D. and Barclay, L. (1997) *Constructing Fatherhood: Discourses and Experiences*. London: Sage.

MacAllister, F. (1995) *Marital Breakdown and the Health of the Nation*, 2nd edn. London: One Plus One Marriage and Partnership Research Charity.

McGleenan, T. (1998) Genetics and insurance: recent developments in the UK, *Euroscreen*, 9: spring.

McHoul, A. and Grace, W. (1993) *A Foucault Primer: Discourse, Power and the Subject.* London: University College London Press.

McIntosh, M. (1996) Social anxieties about lone motherhood and ideologies of the family: two sides of the same coin, in E. Bortolaia Silva (ed.) *Good Enough Mothering? Feminist Perspectives on Lone Motherhood.* London: Routledge.

MacIntyre, S. (1977) Childbirth: the myth of the golden age, *World Medicine,* 15 June: 17–22.

MacKeith, P. (1985) Report of the education and practice working party: a move in the right direction? *Association of Radical Midwives Newsletter,* 26: 6–8.

McNay, L. (1992) *Foucault and Feminism.* Cambridge: Polity Press.

McNeil, M., Varcoe, I. and Yearley, S. (eds) (1990) *The New Reproductive Technologies.* London: Macmillan.

McRae, S. (1993) *Cohabiting Mothers: Changing Marriage and Motherhood?* London: Policy Studies Institute.

MacSween, M. (1993) *Anorexic Bodies: A Feminist and Sociological Analysis of Anorexia Nervosa.* London: Routledge.

Mander, R. (1987) Why choose midwifery? *Nursing Times,* 83(27): 54–6.

Marshall, H. (1991) The social construction of motherhood: an analysis of childcare and parenting manuals, in A. Phoenix, A. Woollett and E. Lloyd (eds) *Motherhood, Meanings, Practices and Ideologies.* London: Sage.

Marsiglio, W. (ed.) (1995a) *Fatherhood: Contemporary Theory, Research and Social Policy.* London: Sage

Marteau, T., Slack, J., Kidd, J. and Shaw, R. (1992) Presenting a routine screening test in antenatal care: practice observed, *Public Health,* 106: 131–40.

Martin, E. (1990) Science and women's bodies: forms of anthropological knowledge, in M. Jacobus, E. Keller and S. Shuttleworth (eds) *Body Politics: Women, Literature and the Discourse of Science.* London: Routledge.

Martin, E. (1993) *The Woman in the Body: A Cultural Analysis of Reproduction.* Buckingham: Open University Press.

Mason, J. (1994) Gender, care and sensibility in family and kin relationships. Paper presented at British Sociological Association annual conference and subsequently published in J. Holland and L. Adkins (eds) (1996) *Sex, Sensibility and the Gendered Body.* London: Macmillan.

Matus, J. (1995) *Unstable Bodies: Victorian Representations of Sexuality and Maternity.* Manchester: Manchester University Press.

Maynard, M. and Winn, J. (1997) Women, violence and male power, in V. Robinson and D. Richardson (eds) *Introducing Women's Studies,* 2nd edn. London: Macmillan.

Meerabeau, L. (1994) Fertility and reproductive technology, in C. Webb (ed.) *Living Sexuality: Issues for Nursing and Health.* Harrow: Scutari.

Melia, K. (1981) 'Student nurses' accounts of their work and training: a qualitative analysis', unpublished Phd thesis. University of Edinburgh.

Melia, K. (1987) *Learning and Working: The Occupational Socialisation of Nurses.* London: Tavistock.

Mendus, S. (1993) Different voices, still lives: problems in the ethics of care, *Journal of Applied Philosophy,* 10(1): 17–27.

MIDIRS (1986) *MIDIRS Information Pack, 2.* Bristol: MIDIRS.

Midwife, Health Visitor and Community Nurse (editorial) (1986) English National Board for Nursing, Midwifery & Health Visiting calls for more direct entry training for midwives, *Midwife, Health Visitor and Community Nurse,* 22(10): 357.

Midwives' Chronicle & Nursing Notes (editorial) (1986) Direct entry midwifery training initiative, *Midwives Chronicle & Nursing Notes,* 99(186): 267–8.

Midwives Legislation Group (1990a) Rationale for a new midwives act, *ARM Midwifery Matters,* 44(Spring): 12.

Midwives Legislation Group (1990b) *Draft Midwives Bill 1990.* Derby: Association of Radical Midwives.

Midwives Legislation Group (1991) News from the Midwives Legislation Group, *ARM Midwifery Matters*, 49(Summer): 18–19.

Miers, M. (forthcoming) *Gender Issues and Nursing Practice*. London: Macmillan.

Miles, A. (1991) *Women, Health and Medicine*. Buckingham: Open University Press.

Millar, J. (1992) Lone mothers and poverty, in C. Glendinning and J. Millar (eds) *Women and Poverty in Britain in the 1990s*. Hemel Hempstead: Harvester Wheatsheaf.

Millar, J. (1996) Mothers, workers, wives: comparing policy approaches to supporting lone mothers, in E. Bortolaia Silva (ed.) *Good Enough Mothering? Feminist Perspectives on Lone Motherhood*. London: Routledge.

Millet, K. (1977) *Sexual Politics*. London: Virago.

Mirzoeff, N. (1995) *Bodyscape, Art, Modernity and the Ideal Figure*. London: Routledge.

Mitchell, J. (1974) *Psychoanalysis and Feminism*. Harmondsworth: Penguin.

Morgan, M. (1994) Sexuality and disability, in C. Webb (ed.) *Living Sexuality: Issues for Nursing and Health*. Harrow: Scutari.

Morris, J. (ed.) (1992) *Alone Together: Voices of Single Mothers*. London: The Women's Press.

MRC Initiative (1994) at http://www.mrc.ac.uk

Mulkay, M. (1997) *The Embryo Research Debate: Science and the Politics of Reproduction*. Cambridge: Cambridge University Press.

Nakano Glenn, E., Chang, G. and Forcey, L. (eds) (1994) *Mothering, Ideology, Experience and Agency*. London: Routledge.

Newson, K. (1986a) Disputed territory, *Nursing Times*, 82(32): 42–3.

Newson, K. (1986b) The future of midwifery education, in *MIDIRS Information Pack, 1*. Bristol: MIDIRS.

Nolan, M. (1998) Teenage pregnancy: a challenge for the government and nation, *Midwives Journal* 1(5): 152–4.

Nuffield Council on Bioethics (1993) *Genetic Screening: Ethical Issues*. London: HMSO.

O'Brien, M. (1981) *The Politics of Reproduction*. London: Routledge.

O'Connor, M. (1992) Women and birth, a national study of intentional home births in Ireland. Unpublished.

O'Connor, M. (1995) *Birth Tides: Turning Towards Home Birth*. London: Harper-Collins.

O'Driscoll, K. and Meagher, D. (1980) *Active Management of Labour*. London: W.B. Saunders.

Oakley, A. (1974a) *Housewife*. Harmondsworth: Allen Lane.

Oakley, A. (1974b) *The Sociology of Housework*. Oxford: Martin Robertson.

Oakley, A. (1979) *Becoming a Mother*. Oxford: Martin Robertson.

Oakley, A. (1980) *Women Confined*. Oxford: Martin Robertson.

Oakley, A. (1986) *The Captured Womb: A History of the Medical Care of Pregnant Women*, 2nd edn. Oxford: Basil Blackwell.

Oakley, A. (1989) Who cares for women? Science versus love in midwifery today, *Midwives Chronicle and Nursing Notes*, July: 214–21.

Oakley, A. (1992) *Social Support and Motherhood: The Natural History of a Research Project*. Oxford: Blackwell.

Oakley, A. (1994) Giving support in pregnancy: the role of research midwives in a randomized controlled trial, in S. Robinson and A. Thomson (eds) *Midwives, Research & Childbirth*. London: Chapman & Hall.

Oakley, A. and Houd, S. (1990) *Helpers in Childbirth: Midwifery Today*. London: Hemisphere Publishing.

Oakley, A. and Richards, M. (1990) Women's experiences of Caesarean delivery, in J. Garcia, R. Fitzpatrick and M. Richards (eds) *The Politics of Maternity Care: Services for Childbearing Women in Twentieth-Century Britain*. Oxford: Oxford University Press.

Oliver, J. (1983) The caring wife, in J. Finch and D. Groves (eds) *A Labour of Love: Women, Work and Caring*. London: Routledge and Kegan Paul.

Oliver, M. (1990) *The Politics of Disablement*. London: Macmillan.

Overall, C. (1995) Frozen embryos and 'fathers rights': parenthood and decision-making in the cryopreservation of embryos, in J. Callahan (ed.) *Reproduction, Ethics and the Law: Feminist Perspectives*. Bloomington, IN: Indiana University Press.

Pahl, J. (1989) *Money and Marriage*. London: Macmillan.

Parker, R. (1997) The production and purpose of maternal ambivalence in W. Hollway and B. Featherstone (eds) *Mothering and Ambivalence*. London: Routledge.

Pascall, G. (1986) *Social Policy: A Feminist Analysis*. London: Tavistock.

Pateman, C. (1988) *The Sexual Contract*. Oxford: Blackwell.

Payne, S. (1991) *Women, Health and Poverty*. Hemel Hempstead: Harvester Wheatsheaf.

Payne, S. and Walker, J. (1996) *Psychology for Nurses and the Caring Professions*. Buckingham: Open University Press.

Peat Marwick McLintock (1989) *Review of the United Kingdom Council and the Four National Boards for Nursing, Midwifery and Health Visiting*. London: HMSO.

Peretz, E. (1990) A maternity service for England and Wales: local authority maternity care in the inter-war period in Oxfordshire and Tottenham, in J. Garcia, R. Kilpatrick and M. Richards (eds) *The Politics of Maternity Care Services for Childbearing Women in the Twentieth Century*. Oxford: Clarendon Press.

Perry, A. (ed.) (1997) *Nursing: A Knowledge Base for Practice*, 2nd edn. London: Arnold.

Petchesky, R. (1986) *Abortion and Woman's Choice: The State, Sexuality and Reproductive Freedom*. London: Verso.

Petchesky, R. (1987) Foetal Images: the power of visual culture in the politics of reproduction, in M. Stanworth (ed.) *Reproductive Technologies: Gender, Motherhood and Medicine*. Oxford: Blackwell.

Pfeffer, N. (1993) *The Stork and the Syringe: A Political History of Reproductive Medicine*. Cambridge: Polity Press.

Phillips, T., Schostak, J., Bedford, H. and Leamon, J. (1996) *The Evaluation of Pre-Registration Undergraduate Degrees in Nursing and Midwifery Programmes*. Norwich: University of East Anglia.

Phoenix, A. (1990) Black women and the maternity services, in J. Garcia, R. Fitzpatrick and M. Richards (eds) *The Politics of Maternity Care: Services for Childbearing Women in Twentieth-Century Britain*. Oxford: Oxford University Press.

Phoenix, A. (1991a) Mothers under twenty: outsider and insider views, in A. Phoenix, A. Woollett and E. Lloyd (eds) *Motherhood: Meanings, Practices and Ideologies*. London: Sage.

Phoenix, A. (1991b) *Young Mothers?* Cambridge: Polity Press.

Phoenix, A. (1996) Social constructions of lone motherhood: a case of competing discourses, in E. Bortolaia Silva (ed.) *Good Enough Mothering? Feminist Perspectives on Lone Motherhood*. London: Routledge.

Phoenix, A. and Wollett, A. (1991) Motherhood: social construction, politics and psychology, in A. Phoenix, A. Wollett and E. Lloyd (eds) *Motherhood Meanings, Practices and Ideologies*. London: Sage.

Phoenix, A., Woollett, A. and Lloyd, E. (eds) (1991) *Motherhood: Meanings, Practices and Ideologies*. London: Sage.

Pleck, J. (1987) American fathering in historical perspective, in M. Kimmel (ed.) *Changing Men: New Directions in Research on Men and Masculinity*. London: Sage.

Pope, V. (1987) Project 2000: the midwifery options, in *Nurse Education Today*, 7: 56–8.

Porter, S. (1998) *Social Theory and Nursing Practice*. London: Macmillan.

Radford, N. and Thompson, A. (1988) *Direct Entry: A Preparation for Midwifery Practice*. Guildford: ENB/University of Surrey.

Rafferty, A. (1996) *The Politics of Nursing Knowledge*. London: Routledge.

Ratcliffe, P. (1991) What future for the boards? *Nursing Times*, 87(10): 57–8.

Rich, A. (1980) Compulsory heterosexuality and lesbian existence, *Signs*, 5(4): 631–60.

Rich, A. (1983) Compulsory heterosexuality and lesbian existence, in S. Sintow, C. Stansell and S. Thompson (eds) *Powers of Desire: The Politics of Sexuality*. New York: New York Monthly Review Press.

Rich, A. (1995) *Of Woman Born: Motherhood as Experience and Institution*, 7th edn. London: Virago.

Richards, M. (1993) The new genetics: some issues for social scientists, *Sociology of Health & Illness*, 15(5): 567–86.

Richardson, D. (1993a) *Women, Motherhood and Childrearing*. London: Macmillan.

Richardson, D. (1993b) The Challenge of AIDS, in S. Jackson, K. Atkinson, D. Beddoe *et al.* (eds) *Women's Studies: A Reader*. Hemel Hempstead: Harvester Wheatsheaf.

Richardson, D. (ed.) (1996a) *Theorising Heterosexuality: Telling it Straight*. Buckingham: Open University Press.

Richardson, D. (1996b) Contradictions in discourse: gender, sexuality and HIV/AIDS, in J. Holland and L. Adkins (eds) *Sex, Sensibility and the Gendered Body*. London: Macmillan.

Richardson, D. (1997) Sexuality and feminism, in V. Robinson and D. Richardson (eds) *Introducing Women's Studies*, 2nd end. London: Macmillan.

Richter, A. (1991) Fighting symbols and structures: postmodernism, feminism and women's health, in L. Nencel and P. Pels (eds) *Constructing Knowledge: Authority and Critique in Social Science*. London: Sage.

Robinson, A. (1998) Hard labour: tough choices, *Guardian*, 18 August: 14–15.

Robinson, J. (1997) First class delivery? Auditing the auditors, *British Journal of Midwifery*, 5(4): 227.

Robinson, K. and Vaughan, B. (1993) *Knowledge for Nursing Practice*, 2nd edn. Oxford: Butterworth-Heinemann.

Robinson, S. (1986) Career intentions of newly qualified midwives, *Midwifery*, 3: 25–36.

Robinson, S. (1990) Maintaining the independence of midwives, in J. Garcia, R. Kilpatrick and M. Richards (eds) *The Politics of Maternity Care Services for Childbearing Women in Twentieth-Century Britain*. Oxford: Oxford University Press.

Roch, S. (1986) Project 2000: the way forward for midwives, *Midwives Chronicle & Nursing Notes*, 99: 21–4.

Rose, H. (1994) *Love, Power and Knowledge: Towards a Feminist Transformation of the Sciences*. Cambridge: Polity Press.

Roseneil, S. and Mann, K. (1996) Unpalatable choices and inadequate families, lone mothers and the underclass debate, in R. Bortolaia Silva (ed.) *Good Enough Mothering? Feminist Perspectives on Lone Motherhood*. London: Routledge.

Rowland, R. (1993) *Living Laboratories: Women and Reproductive Technology*, 2nd edn. London: Cedar.

Royal College of Midwives (1986) *Comments of the RCM on UKCC Project 2000*. London: RCM.

Royal College of Midwives (1987) *The Role and Education of the Future Midwife in the United Kingdom*. London: RCM.

Royal College of Midwives (1991) *Report of the Royal College of Midwives' Commission on Legislation Relating to Midwives*. London: RCM.

Royal College of Midwives (1993) *Guidelines for the Provision of Midwifery Education*. London: RCM.

Royal College of Midwives (date unknown) *The Midwife: Her Legal Status and Her Accountability*. London: RCM.

Royal College of Nursing (1985) *Commission on Nursing Education: The Education of Nurses, a New Dispensation*. London: RCN.

Royal College of Obstetricians & Gynaecologists (1992) *Response of the RCOG to the Report of the House of Commons Committee on Maternity Services*. London: RCOG.

Royal College of Physicians (1989) *Prenatal Diagnosis and Genetic Screening: Community Service Implications*. London: RCOP.

Royal College of Physicians (1990) *Teaching Genetics to Medical Students: A Survey and Recommendations*. London: RCOP.

Ruddick, S. (1982) Maternal thinking, in B. Thorne and M. Yalom (eds) *Rethinking the Family*. London: Longman.

Safe Motherhood (1996) Early sex, early motherhood: facing the challenge, *Safe Motherhood Newsletter*, 22(3): 4–8.

Saffron, L. (1994) *Challenging Conceptions*. London: Cassell.

Salvage, J. and Kershaw, B. (eds) (1990) *Models for Nursing 2*. Harrow: Scutari.

Sandall, J. (1995) Choice, continuity and control: a sociological perspective, *Midwifery*, 11: 201–9.

Sandall, J. (1996) Continuity of midwifery care in Britain: a new professional project, *Gender, Work and Organisation*, 3(4): 215–26.

Sandall, J. (1997) Midwives' burnout and continuity of care, *British Journal of Midwifery*, 5(2): 106–11.

Saranga, E. (ed.) (1998) *Embodying the Social: Constructions of Difference*. London: Routledge.

Savage, J. (1987) *Nurses, Gender and Sexuality*. London: Heinemann.

Savage, W. (1988) *A Savage Inquiry: Who Controls Childbirth?* 2nd edn. London: Virago.

Savage, W. (1990) How obstetricians might change, in J. Garcia, R. Fitzpatrick and M. Richards (eds) *The Politics of Maternity Care: Services for Childbearing Women in Twentieth-Century Britain*. Oxford: Oxford University Press.

Sawicki, J. (1991) *Disciplining Foucault: Feminism, Power and the Body*. London: Routledge.

Schön, D. (1983) *The Reflective Practitioner: How Professionals Think in Action*. New York: Basic Books.

Schön, D. (1987) *Educating the Reflective Practitioner*. London: Jossey Bass.

Schwarz, E. (1990) The engineering of childbirth in J. Garcia, R. Fitzpatrick and M. Richards (eds) *The Politics of Maternity Care: Services for Childbearing Women in Twentieth-Century Britain*. Oxford: Oxford University Press.

Scott, J. (1992) Experience, in J. Butler and J. Scott (eds) *Feminists Theorize the Political*. London: Routledge.

Scott, S. and Morgan, D. (eds) (1993) *Body Matters: Essays on the Sociology of the Body*. London: Falmer Press.

Scruggs, M. (1986) Project 2000 and the midwife: grasping the nettle, *Midwives' Chronicle and Nursing Notes*, 99: 214–15.

Segal, L. (1990) *Slow Motion: Changing Masculinities, Changing Men*. London: Virago.

Segal, L. (1995) A feminist looks at the family, in J. Muncie, M. Wetherell, R. Dallos and A. Cochrane (eds) *Understanding the Family*. London: Open University/Sage.

Segal, L. (1997) Sexualities, in K. Woodward (ed.) *Identity and Difference*. London: Sage.

Shanley, M. (1995) Fathers' rights, mothers' wrongs? Reflections on unwed fathers' rights, patriarchy and sex equality, in J. Callahan (ed.) *Reproduction, Ethics and the Law: Feminist Perspectives*. Bloomington, IN: Indiana University Press.

Shickle, D. and Chadwick, R. (1994) The ethics of screening: is 'screeningitis' an incurable disease? *Journal of Medical Ethics*, 20: 12–18.

Shildrick, M. (1997) *Leaky Bodies and Boundaries: Feminism, Postmodernism and (Bio)ethics*. London: Routledge.

Shilling, C. (1993) *The Body and Social Theory*. London: Sage.

Shilling, C. (1997) The body and difference, in K. Woodward (ed.) *Identity and Difference*. London: Sage.

Silverton, L. (1996) Educating for the future, in D. Kroll (ed.) *Midwifery Care for the Future, Meeting the Challenge*. London: Bailliere Tindall.

Simpson, I. (1979) *From Student to Nurse: A Longitudinal Study of Socialisation*. Cambridge: Cambridge University Press.

Sleep, J. (1995) Changing practice through research, in *Changing Childbirth Educational Resource Pack for Midwives no. 2: Choice for the Midwife*. London: ENB.

Smart, C. (1987) There is of course a distinction dictated by nature: law and the problem of paternity, in M. Stanworth (ed.) *Reproductive Technologies: Gender, Motherhood and Medicine*. Oxford: Blackwell.

Smart, C. (1996) Deconstructing motherhood, in E. Bortolaia Silva (ed.) *Good Enough Mothering? Feminist Perspectives on Lone Motherhood*. London: Routledge.

Smart, C. (1997) Desperately seeking post-heterosexual woman, in J. Holland and L. Adkins (eds) *Sex, Sensibility and the Gendered Body*. London: Macmillan.

Spallone, P. (1989) *Beyond Conception: The New Politics of Reproduction*. London: Macmillan.

Spallone, P. (1992) *Generation Games: Genetic Engineering and the Future of Our Lives*. Philadelphia: Temple University Press.

Spelman, E. (1988) *Inessential Woman: Problems of Exclusion in Feminist Thought*. Boston, MA: Beacon Press.

Spence, J. (1986) *Putting Myself in the Picture*. London: Camden Press.

Spence, J. (1995) *Cultural Sniping: The Art of Transgression*. London: Routledge.

Stacey, J. (1997) Feminist theory: capital F, capital T, in V. Robinson and D. Richardson (eds) *Introducing Women's Studies*, 2nd edn. London: Macmillan.

Stacey, M. (ed.) (1992) *Changing Human Reproduction: Social Science Perspectives*. London: Sage.

Stanley, L. and Wise, S. (1993) *Breaking Out Again: Feminist Ontology and Epistemology*. London: Routledge.

Stanworth, M. (ed.) (1987) *Reproductive Technologies: Gender, Motherhood and Medicine*. Cambridge: Polity Press.

Starkey, F. (1998) Maternity and health links: an advocacy service for Asian women and their families, in L. Doyal (ed.) *Women and Health Services*. Buckingham: Open University Press.

Statham, H. (1994) The parents' reaction to termination of pregnancy for fetal abnormality: from a mother's point of view, in L. Abramsky and J. Chapple (eds) *Prenatal Diagnosis. The Human Side*. London: Chapman & Hall.

Statham, H. and Green, J. (1993) Serum screening for Down's syndrome: some women's experiences, *British Medical Journal*, 307: 174–6.

Stern, P. (1993) *Lesbian Health: What are the issues?* London: Taylor & Francis.

Strong, P. and Robinson, J. (1990) *The NHS: Under New Management*. Buckingham: Open University Press.

Symon, A. (1995) Professional and legal accountability: how it will be influenced by *Changing Childbirth* recommendations, in *Changing Childbirth Educational Resource Pack for Midwives, no. 4: Control in Practice*. London: ENB.

Symonds, A. and Hunt, S. (1996) *The Midwife and Society: Perspectives, Policies and Practice*. London: Macmillan.

Tew, M. (1992) *Safer Childbirth? A Critical History of Maternity Care*. London: Chapman & Hall.

Tew, M. (1995) *Safer Childbirth? A Critical History of Maternity Care*, 2nd edn. London: Chapman & Hall.

Thomas, J. (1979) ARM's campaign against the bill, *Association of Radical Midwives Newsletter*, February: 8–9.

Thomas, H. (1998) Reproductive needs across the lifespan, in L. Doyal (ed.) *Women and Health Services*. Buckingham: Open University Press.

Thornley, C. (1996) Segmentation and inequality in the nursing workforce: re-evaluating the evaluation of skills, in R. Crompton, D. Gallie and K. Purcell (eds) *Changing Forms of Employment Organisations, Skills and Gender*. London: Routledge.

Tickner, V. (1986) On the Right Lines But . . . , *Senior Nurse*, 5(5/6): 34–6.

Tilsey, L. (1997) Sexual health and teenagers, *Practice Nurse*, 13(9): 541–4.

Tizard, B. (1991) Employed mothers and the care of young children, in A. Pheonix, A. Woollett and E. Lloyd (eds) *Motherhood, Meanings, Practices and Ideologies*. London: Sage.

Tong, R. (1992) *Feminist Thought: An Introduction*. London: Routledge.

Towler, J. and Bramall, J. (1986) *Midwives in History and Society*. London: Croom Helm.

Tronto, J. (1993) *Moral Boundaries: A Political Argument for an Ethic of Care*. London: Routledge.

Turner, B. (1992) *Regulating Bodies: Essays in Medical Sociology*. London: Routledge.

Turner, B. (1995) *Medical Knowledge and Social Power*. London: Sage.

Turney, J. (1995) The public understanding of genetics: where next? *European Journal Genetics Society*, 1: 5–20.

Turton, P. (1994) Community care for people living with HIV/AIDS, in C. Webb (ed.) *Living Sexuality: Issues for Nursing and Health*. Harrow: Scutari.

UKCC (United Kingdom Central Council for Nursing, Midwifery and Health Visiting) (1986a) *Project 2000: A New Preparation for Practice*. London: UKCC.

UKCC (United Kingdom Central Council for Nursing, Midwifery and Health Visiting) (1986b) *Project 2000 and the Midwife*. London: UKCC.

UKCC (United Kingdom Central Council for Nursing, Midwifery and Health Visiting) (1991a) *Midwives' Rules*. London: UKCC.

UKCC (United Kingdom Central Council for Nursing, Midwifery and Health Visiting) (1991b) *A Midwife's Code of Practice*. London: UKCC.

UKCC (United Kingdom Central Council for Nursing, Midwifery and Health Visiting) (1998) The future of professional regulation. UKCC website entry.

Ungerson, C. (ed.) (1990) *Gender and Caring*. Hemel Hempstead: Harvester Wheatsheaf.

Utting, D. (1995) *Family and Parenthood: Supporting Families, Preventing Breakdown*. York: Joseph Rowntree Foundation.

VanEvery, J. (1995) *Heterosexual Women Changing the Family: Refusing to be a 'Wife'!* London: Taylor & Francis.

Versluyen, M. (1981) Midwives, medical men and 'poor women labouring of child': lying-in hospitals in eighteenth-century London, in H. Roberts (ed.) *Women, Health and Reproduction*. London: Routledge and Kegan Paul.

Walby, S. (1986) *Patriarchy at Work*. Oxford: Polity Press.

Walby, S. (1990) *Theorising Patriarchy*. Oxford: Blackwell.

Walby, S. and Greenwell, J. with Mackay, L. and Soothill, K. (1994) *Medicine and Nursing*. London: Sage.

Waldby, C. (1996) *AIDS and the Body Politic, Biomedicine and Sexual Difference*. London: Routledge.

Walpin, L. (1997) Combating heterosexism: implications for nursing, *Clinical Nurse Specialist*, 11(3): 126–32.

Walsh, D. and Crompton, A. (1997) A review of midwifery-led care: some challenges and constraints, *MIDIRS Midwifery Digest*, 7(1): 113–17.

Walton, I. (1994) *Sexuality and Motherhood*. Oxford: Butterworth-Heinemann.

Walton, I. and Hamilton, M. (1995) *Midwives and Changing Childbirth*. Hale: Royal College of Midwives and Books for Midwives Press.

Warnock, M. (1985) *A Question of Life: The Warnock Report on Human Fertilization and Embryology*. Oxford: Blackwell.

Warwick, C. (1992) Reflections on the current management of midwifery education, *Midwifery*, 2(2): 251–4.

Waterhouse, J. (1996) Nursing practice related to sexuality: a review and recommendations, *NT Research*, 1(6): 412–18.

Waters, J. (1996) High hopes, *Nursing Times*, 92(42): 16–17.

Weatherall, D. (1991) *The New Genetics and Clinical Practice*. Oxford: Oxford University Press.

Webb, C. (1985) *Sexuality, Nursing and Health*. Chichester: Wiley.

Webb, C. (ed.) (1994) *Living Sexuality: Issues for Nursing and Health*. Harrow: Scutari.

Webb, W. (1994) Teen sexuality: empowering teens to decide, *Policy Studies Review*, 13(1–2): 127–40.

Webster, A. (1991) *Science, Technology and Society*. London: Macmillan.

Weeks, J. (1981) *Sex, Politics and Society. The Regulation of Sexuality Since 1800*. Harlow: Longman.

Weeks, J. (1985) *Sexuality and its Discontents. Meanings, Myths and Modern Sexualities*. London: Routledge and Kegan Paul.

Weeks, J. (1986) *Sexuality*. London: Tavistock.

Weeks, J. (1991) *Against Nature: Essays on History, Sexuality and Identity*. London: Rivers Oram Press.

Weeks, J. (1994) *The Lesser Evil and the Greater Good*. London: Rivers Oram Press.

Westwood, S. (1996) 'Feckless fathers': masculinities and the British state, in M. Mac An Ghaill (ed.) *Understanding Masculinities*. Buckingham: Open University Press.

Wetherell, M. (1995) The psychoanalytic approach to family life, in J. Muncie, M. Wetherell, R. Dallos and A. Cochrane (eds) *Understanding the Family*. London: Open University/Sage.

Whitehead, M. (1988) *The Health Divide: Inequalities in Health in the 1980s*. Harmondsworth: Penguin.

Whitford, M. (1991) *Luce Irigaray: Philosopher in the Feminine*. London: Routledge.

Wilkinson, S. and Kitzenger, C. (eds) (1993a) *Heterosexuality: A Reader*. London: Sage.

Wilkinson, S. and Kitzinger, C. (eds) (1993b) *Heterosexuality: A Feminism and Psychology Reader*. London: Sage.

Williams, S. and Calnan, M. (eds) (1996) *Modern Medicine: Lay Perspectives and Experiences*. London: University College London Press.

Wilton, T. (1995) *Lesbian Studies: Setting An Agenda*. London: Routledge.

Wilton, T. (1997) *Good For You: A Handbook on Lesbian Health and Wellbeing*. London: Cassell.

Wilton, T. (1998) Gender, sexuality and healthcare: improving services, in L. Doyal (ed.) *Women and Health Services*. Buckingham: Open University Press.

Winslade, W. (1981) Surrogate mothers: private right or public wrong? *Journal of Medical Ethics*, 7: 153–4.

Witz, A. (1992) *Professions and Patriarchy*. London: Routledge.

Woodward, K. (ed.) (1997) *Identity and Difference*. London: Sage and the Open University.

Woolgar, S. (1988) *Science: The Very Idea*. London: Tavistock.

Young, I. (1984) Pregnant embodiment: subjectivity and alienation, *Journal of Medicine and Philosophy*, 9: 45–62.

Young, I. (1990) *Throwing Like a Girl and Other Essays in Feminist Philosophy and Social Theory*. Bloomington, IN: Indiana University Press.

INDEX